MILADY'S STANDARD
COSMETOLOGY
PRACTICAL
WORKBOOK

MILADY'S STANDARD
COSMETOLOGY
PRACTICAL
WORKBOOK

To be used with
MILADY'S STANDARD COSMETOLOGY

Compiled by
Catherine Frangie

THOMSON

DELMAR LEARNING AUSTRALIA CANADA MEXICO SINGAPORE SPAIN UNITED KINGDOM UNITED STATES

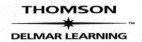

THOMSON
™
DELMAR LEARNING

Milady's Standard Cosmetology Practical Workbook

Library of Congress Catalog Card Number: 2002074216
ISBN 1-56253-891-8

NOTICE TO THE READER

Publisher does not warrant or guarantee any of the products described herein or perform any independent analysis in connection with any of the product information contained herein. Publisher does not assume, and expressly disclaims, any obligation to obtain and include information other than that provided to it by the manufacturer.

The reader is expressly warned to consider and adopt all safety precautions that might be indicated by the activities herein and to avoid all potential hazards. By following the instructions contained herein, the reader willingly assumes all risks in connection with such instructions.

The Publisher makes no representation or warranties of any kind, including but not limited to, the warranties of fitness for particular purpose or merchantability, nor are any such representations implied with respect to the material set forth herein, and the publisher takes no responsibility with respect to such material. The publisher shall not be liable for any special, consequential, or exemplary damages resulting, in whole or part, from the readers' use of, or reliance upon, this material.

CONTENTS

How to Use This Workbook

Milady's Standard Cosmetology Practical Workbook has been written to meet the needs, interests, and abilities of students receiving training in cosmetology.

This workbook should be used together with *Milady's Standard Cosmetology* and *Milady's Standard Cosmetology Theory Workbook*. This book directly follows the theoretical information found in the student textbook. Pages to be read and studied are listed at the beginning of each chapter. The theory information can be found in *Milady's Standard Cosmetology Theory Workbook*.

Students are to answer each item in this workbook with a pencil after consulting their textbook for correct information. Items can be corrected and/or rated during class or individual discussions, or on an independent study basis.

Various tests are included to emphasize essential facts found in the textbook and to measure the student's progress.

1

COSMETOLOGY: THE HISTORY AND OPPORTUNITIES

See Milady's Standard Cosmetology Theory Workbook

2

LIFE SKILLS

See Milady's Standard Cosmetology Theory Workbook

3

YOUR PROFESSIONAL IMAGE

See Milady's Standard Cosmetology Theory Workbook

4

COMMUNICATING FOR SUCCESS

See Milady's Standard Cosmetology Theory Workbook

5

INFECTION CONTROL: PRINCIPLES AND PRACTICE

Date: _____
Rating:_____
Text Pages: 93-127

POINT TO PONDER:

"Learning makes a man fit company for himself."—Young

PRINCIPLES OF PREVENTION

1. What is the best way for a salon to make a good first impression?

   _____

   _____

2. In the salon proper care must be taken to meet rigorous _____ , otherwise

   the salon could be contributing to the spread of disease.

   a) food and drug standards

   b) technical standards

   c) health standards

   d) temperature standards

3. Controlling_____is a vitally important aspect of the salon industry

   because clients depend upon you to ensure their safety.

4. Surfaces of tools or other objects that are not free from dirt, oils, and microbes are covered with

   _____ , which are any substances that can cause contamination.

5. List some of the things in the salon that can be contaminants.

   a) _____

   b) _____

   c) _____

6. Tools and other surfaces in the salon that look clean can be contaminated with bacteria, viruses, and fungi.

   _____ True

   _____ False

7. The removal of pathogens and other substances from tools and surfaces is called _____.

8. Decontamination involves the use of _____ or _____ means to remove, inactivate, or destroy pathogens so that the object is rendered safe for handling, use, or disposal.

9. What are the three main levels of decontamination?

   a) _____

   b) _____

   c) _____

10. Are all three levels of decontamination required in the salon?

    _____

11. _____ is the highest level of decontamination.

12. Sterilization does not completely destroy every organism on a surface, whether beneficial or harmful.

    _____ True

    _____ False

13. What are the methods of sterilization?

    _____

14. _____ use needles and probes that lance the skin, so they must follow the same sterilization procedures as doctors and surgeons.

15. _____ are a simpler solution to the issue of sterilization.

16. _____ is the second highest level of decontamination.

17. The difference between disinfection and sterilization is:

_____

18. Disinfection controls _____ on hard, nonporous surfaces such as cuticle

nippers and other salon implements.

19. _____ are chemical agents used to destroy most bacteria and disinfect implements.

20. Disinfectants are for use on:

a) human skin

b) hair

c) combs

d) fingernails

21. Why should you never use disinfectants as hand cleaners?

_____

_____

22. Like all tools, disinfectants must always be used in strict accordance with _____

_____.

23. All disinfectants must be approved by the _____

and each individual state.

24. The disinfectant's label must also have a/an _____

which ensures that the EPA has the necessary test data on file and that the product has been proven

effective against certain organisms.

25. The_____ will also tell you exactly which organisms the disinfectant has

been tested for, such as HIV-1 and the Hepatitis B Virus.

26. The_____ provides all pertinent information on

products, ranging from content and associated hazards to combustion levels and storage requirements.

27. What does OSHA stand for, and what is it?

    _____

    _____

28. To meet salon requirements, a disinfectant must have the correct_____ to be used

    against bacteria, fungi, and viruses.

29. A disinfectant that is "Formulated for Hospitals and Health Care Facilities" or a "Hospital Disinfectant"
    must be:

    a) _____

    b) _____

    c) _____

    d) _____

30. When salon implements accidentally come into contact with blood or body fluids, how should they be
    treated?

    _____

    _____

31. Any item that is used on a client must be _____ or _____ after each use.

32. Before implements are soaked in a disinfecting solution, they should be:

    _____

33. Implements must be _____ submerged for proper disinfection.

    a) partially

    b) halfway

    c) two-thirds

    d) completely

34. _____ use high-frequency sound waves to create powerful cleansing bubbles

    in the liquid that clean tiny crevices that are impossible to reach with a brush.

35. Match the following types of disinfectants with their descriptions:

    _____ 1. quats   A. caustic poison

    _____ 2. phenol   B. nontoxic, odorless, and fast acting disinfectant

    _____ 3. isopropyl alcohol   C. effective and readily available disinfectant, is also known as bleach

    _____ 4. sodium hypochlorite   D. 99% solution strength disinfectant

36. What are quats?

_____

_____

37. Most quat solutions disinfect implements in_____ minutes.

    a) 5 to 10

    b) 10 to 15

    c) 15 to 20

    d) 25 to 30

38. List the safety precautions to take when using disinfectants.

    a) _____

       _____

    b) _____

       _____

    c) _____

       _____

    d) _____

       _____

    e) _____

       _____

    f) _____

       _____

    g) _____

       _____

    h) _____

       _____

39. What is a wet sanitizer?

_____

40. List the steps involved in disinfecting tools and implements such as combs, brushes, rollers, picks, styling tools, scissors, tweezers, nail clippers, and some nail files.

   a) _____

   _____

   b) _____

   _____

   c) _____

   _____

   d) _____

   _____

   e) _____

   _____

   f) _____

   _____

   g) _____

   _____

   h) _____

   _____

41. How should you disinfect salon linens and capes?

_____

_____

42. How should electrical equipment be disinfected?

_____

_____

_____

43. How should work surfaces be disinfected?

_____

_____

44. How should the shampoo bowl be disinfected?

_____

_____

_____

45. How should whirlpool pedicure foot spas be handled after each client?

a) _____

_____

b) _____

_____

c) _____

_____

d) _____

_____

46. How should whirlpool pedicure foot spas be handled at the end of each day?

a) _____

_____

b) _____

_____

_____

c) _____

_____

d) _____

_____

47. How should whirlpool pedicure foot spas be handled every two weeks?

a) _____

b) _____

c) _____

d) _____

48. How should a blood spill in the salon be handled?

a) _____

b) _____

c) _____

d) _____

e) _____

f) _____

g) _____

h) _____

i) _____

j) _____

_____

_____

49. The _____ must be kept clean and orderly, with all containers marked clearly as to

content. A/an _____ on every chemical in stock should be kept readily available to all

those working in the salon or school.

50. How should contaminated disposable supplies be thrown away?

_____

_____

51. The third, or lowest, level of decontamination is _____.

52. To sanitize means to _____

_____.

53. _____ is a fungus growth that usually grows in dark, damp places. _____ is a moldy coating produced by fungi that can appear on walls, fabrics, and the like and also occurs in damp areas.

54. List the steps for washing your hands.

a) _____

b) _____

_____

_____

c) _____

d) _____

55. _____ can kill, retard, or prevent the growth of bacteria, but they are not classified as disinfectants.

56. Antiseptics are _____ than disinfectants and are _____ for application to skin.

57. For each of the following, note in the space next to it whether the item must be sterilized, disinfected or sanitized for use in the salon.

lancets   _____

combs and brushes   _____

shampoo bowls   _____

Velcro rollers   _____

haircutting shears   _____

UNIVERSAL PRECAUTIONS

58. Why should you use the same infection control practices with all clients?

_____

_____

59. _____ are a set of guidelines and controls, published by the Centers for

Disease Control and Prevention (CDC), that require the employer and the employee to assume that all

human blood and specified human body fluids are infectious for HIV, HBV, and other bloodborne

pathogens.

60. Universal precautions include:

_____

_____

_____

61. List all of the guidelines you should follow to keep your salon looking its best and being its best:

a) _____

b) _____

c) _____

d) _____

e) _____

f) _____

g) _____

h) _____

i) _____

j) _____

k) _____

l) _____

m) _____

n) _____

o) _____

p) _____

q) _____

r) _____

s) _____

t) _____

u) _____

_____

v) _____

w) _____

x) _____

_____

y) _____

_____

_____

z) _____

6

ANATOMY AND PHYSIOLOGY

See Milady's Standard Cosmetology Theory Workbook

7

BASICS OF CHEMISTRY AND ELECTRICITY

See Milady's Standard Cosmetology Theory Workbook

8

PROPERTIES OF THE HAIR AND SCALP

See Milady's Standard Cosmetology Theory Workbook

9

PRINCIPLES OF HAIR DESIGN

See Milady's Standard Cosmetology Theory Workbook

10
SHAMPOOING, RINSING, & CONDITIONING

Date: _____

Rating: _____

Text Pages: 255-279

POINT TO PONDER:

"The best teacher is the one who suggests rather than dogmatizes, and inspires the listener with the wish to teach himself."—Bulwer

SCALP MASSAGE

1. The two basic requisites for a healthy scalp are _____ and _____

2. Scalp manipulations should be given with a _____ motion, which will _____

   _____ .

3. Scalp massage is most effective when given as a series of treatments— _____

   for a normal scalp and _____ when scalp disorders are present, in conjunction

   with treatment by a dermatologist.

4. Scalp massage is performed _____ the shampoo.

   a) after

   b) before

   c) during

   d) throughout

5. When giving a scalp massage, what parts of your hands will be in use, and what will they be stimulating?

   _____

   _____

6. Describe how the relaxing movement is performed.

7. Describe how the sliding movement is performed.

8. Describe how the sliding and rotating movement is performed.

9. Describe how the forehead movement is performed.

10. Describe how the scalp movement is performed.

11. Describe how the hairline movement is performed.

12. Describe how the front scalp movement is performed.

13. Describe how the back scalp movement is performed.

   _____

   _____

   _____

14. Describe how the ear-to-ear movement is performed.

   _____

   _____

15. Describe how the back movement is performed.

   _____

   _____

   _____

16. Describe how the front shoulder movement is performed.

   _____

   _____

   _____

17. Describe how the spine movement is performed.

   _____

   _____

THE SHAMPOO PROCEDURE

18. Why is it important for you to maintain good posture while performing a shampoo?

   _____

   _____

19. What is the most important rule to remember regarding posture?

   _____

   _____

20. What types of shampoo bowls allow for healthier body alignment and help reduce strain on the back and shoulders?

   _____

21. What are the implements and materials you will need to perform a basic shampoo?

   a) _____   d) _____

   b) _____   e) _____

   c) _____

22. What three things should you do before draping the client for a shampoo?

   a) _____

   b) _____

   c) _____

23. How do you drape a client for the shampoo?

   a) _____

   b) _____

   c) _____

   _____

   d) _____

24. How should you prepare the hair and the client before the shampoo?

   a) _____

   b) _____

   c) _____

   _____

   d) _____

   e) _____

25. How should you seat the client comfortably at the shampoo bowl?

   _____

   _____

26. What temperature of water is best for shampooing?

    a) hot

    b) cold

    c) warm

    d) freezing

27. How should you test the water temperature?

    _____

28. Where should one finger be during the entire shampoo and why?

    _____

    _____

    _____

29. What is the best way to wet the hair thoroughly?

    _____

30. How should you work around the hairline to protect the client's face, ears, and neck from the spray?

    _____

    _____

31. Where should you begin the shampoo?

    _____

    _____

32. When shampooing, you must use your fingernails in the clients scalp in order to give a good scalp manipulation.

    _____ True

    _____ False

33. What is the procedure for manipulating the scalp?

    a) _____

    _____

b) _____

_____

c) _____

_____

d) _____

_____

e) _____

_____

f) _____

_____

g) _____

_____

h) _____

_____

34. Describe how to rinse hair thoroughly to remove all of the shampoo lather.

_____

_____

_____

35. List the steps involved in applying a conditioner to shampooed hair.

a) _____

_____

b) _____

_____

c) _____

_____

d) _____

_____

e) _____

_____

36. If the conditioner you've applied is to remain on the head for more than one minute, what position should the client be in for her comfort?

_____

_____

_____

37. Once the conditioner is rinsed out, you should

_____   a)   blow-dry the hair

_____   b)   partially towel-dry the hair

_____   c)   comb out the hair

_____   d)   brush through the hair

38. Describe how to partially towel-dry the hair.

a) _____

b) _____

c) _____

d) _____

39. Should you ever rub the hair with the towel? Why or why not?

_____

40. After the shampoo, you should _____ the shampoo bowl, removing any _____.

41. Once the client is back at your station you should _____, beginning with

the ends at the nape of the neck.

42. If the drape is wet, what should you do?

_____

43. How should you clean up after the shampoo?

    a) _____

    b) _____

    c) _____

    d) _____

    e) _____

44. Why does chemically treated hair require special care during the shampoo process?

    _____

45. What kind of shampoo is best for chemically treated hair?

    _____

46. If chemically treated hair becomes tangled, how should you treat it?

    _____

    _____

47. How is a dry shampoo applied?

    _____

    _____

48. How should you care for and service disabled or wheelchair-bound clients?

    _____

    _____

49. What are some options for shampooing a client in a wheelchair?

    _____

    _____

    _____

GENERAL HAIR AND SCALP TREATMENTS

50. The purpose of a general scalp treatment is to keep the scalp and hair in a _____ and _____ condition.

51. A stylist should recommend a hair or scalp treatment only after having performed a _____ _____ .

52. List the steps involved in performing normal hair and scalp treatments.

    a) _____

    b) _____

    c) _____

    d) _____

    e) _____

    f) _____

    g) _____

    h) _____

    i) _____

53. If you find a client has a deficiency of natural oil on the scalp and hair, you should select scalp preparations containing _____ and _____ ingredients.

54. What should you avoid using on dry scalps?

    a) _____

    b) _____

    c) _____

    d) _____

55. List the steps involved in performing dry hair and scalp treatments.

    a) _____

    b) _____

    c) _____

d) _____

_____

e) _____

f) _____

g) _____

h) _____

_____

i) _____

j) _____

56. Excessive oiliness is caused by overactive _____ glands.

57. How should you manipulate the scalp to increase blood circulation to the surface?

_____

58. What else will happen as a result of kneading the scalp?

_____

_____

59. List the steps involved in performing oily hair and scalp treatments.

a) _____

b) _____

c) _____

d) _____

e) _____

f) _____

g) _____

h) _____

i) _____

j) _____

60. What procedure should you follow if you need to treat a scalp with a dandruff condition?

a) _____

b) _____

c) _____

d) _____

e) _____

f) _____

g) _____

h) _____

i) _____

j) _____

11

HAIRCUTTING

Date: _____

Rating: _____

Text Pages: 281-345

POINT TO PONDER:

"Wisdom is the right use of knowledge. To know is not to be wise. Many men know a great deal, and are all the greater fools for it. There is no fool so great as a knowing fool. But to know how to use knowledge is to have wisdom."—Spurgeon

BASIC PRINCIPLES OF HAIRCUTTING

1. Understanding the physics of hair means that for every action or technique you use on the hair, there

   will be an _____ and _____ result.

2. The shape of the head or skull, also referred to as the _____ or _____,

   plays a major role in guiding you to the desired result.

3. What is a reference point?

   _____

   _____

4. List some commonly used reference points.

   _____

5. Why are reference points used?

   a) _____

   b) _____

   c) _____

   _____

6. Match the following reference points with their descriptions.

_____ 1. parietal ridge   A. the back corner of the head

_____ 2. occipital bone   B. the widest area of the head, starts at temples, ends at bottom of the crown

_____ 3. apex   C. the bone that protrudes at the base of the skull

_____ 4. four corners   D. the highest point on the top of the head

7. How can you find/determine the parietal ridge?

_____

_____

8. How can you find/determine the occipital bone?

_____

9. How can you find/determine the apex?

_____

10. How can you find/determine the four corners?

_____

_____

_____

11. Where is the top of the head and why is it important to identify?

_____

_____

12. Where is the front of the head?

_____

_____

_____

13. Where are the sides of the head?

_____

14. Where is the crown and why is it important to identify?

_____

_____

15. Where is the nape?

_____

16. Where is the back of the head?

_____

_____

17. Where is the fringe or bangs area?

_____

18. A line is the space between two lines or surfaces that intersect at a given point.

_____ True

_____ False

19. An angle is the space between _____.

20. Two basic lines used in haircutting are:

_____ a)   straight and round

_____ b)   straight and curved

_____ c)   straight and diagonal

_____ d)   diagonal and curved

21. Label the three types of straight lines illustrated below.

1. _____

2. _____

3 _____

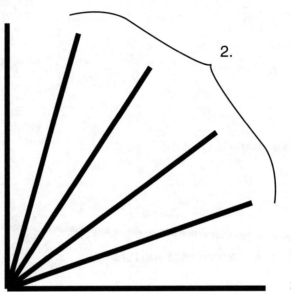

1.

2.

3.

22. Horizontal lines are used to create _____ and _____ haircuts because

    they _____ .

23. Vertical lines are usually used to create _____ and _____ haircuts and are used

    with _____ elevations because vertical lines _____ .

24. Diagonal lines are used to create _____ and to _____ .

25. What is beveling?

    _____

26. Why are angles important in haircutting?

    _____

27. The hair is parted into uniform working areas, called _____ , for control during haircutting.

    Each section is further divided into smaller parts called _____ .

28. Elevation is the _____

    _____ .

29. In a blunt or one-length haircut, what degree of elevation is employed?

    _____ a) 90

    _____ b) 45

    _____ c) 30

    _____ d) 0

30. When you elevate the hair below 90 degrees, you are:

    _____ a) removing weight

    _____ b) building weight

    _____ c) removing bulk

    _____ d) thinning hair

31. The _____ is the angle at which the fingers are held when cutting, and ultimately the line that is cut.

32. What is a guideline?

    _____

    _____

33. A guideline that does not move is called a _____ guide.

34. A guide that moves as the haircut progresses is called a _____ guideline.

35. What is overdirection and why is it used?

    _____

    _____

    _____

CLIENT CONSULTATION

36. During the client consultation, before cutting the hair, you will want to examine the following:

a) _____

d) _____

b) _____

e) _____

c) _____

f) _____

37. Weight and volume in a finished hairstyle will _____ attention to an area.

    a) draw

    b) detract

38. _____ is the number of individual hair strands on one square inch of scalp and is usually described as thin, medium, or thick.

39. _____ is the diameter of the hair strands and is usually classified as coarse, medium, and fine.

40. Why are density and texture important?

    _____

    _____

41. The _____ is the amount of movement in the hair strand and is usually classified as straight, wavy, curly, extremely curly, or anything in between.

42. Why are both the hairline and the growth patterns important to examine?

    _____

TOOLS, BODY POSITION, AND SAFETY

43. Match the following tools with their most common use in haircutting.

    _____ 1. haircutting shears   A. used to remove bulk from the hair
    _____ 2. thinning shears   B. used for most haircutting procedures
    _____ 3. straight razor   C. used to keep sections of hair separated from one another
    _____ 4. clippers   D. used for close tapers at nape and sides when using
                                            shears-over-comb technique
    _____ 5. edgers   E. used when creating short tapers, short haircuts, fades,
                                            and flat tops
    _____ 6. styling/cutting comb   F. used when a softer effect is desired on the ends of the hair
    _____ 7. barber comb   G. used to cut blunt or straight lines in hair
    _____ 8. wide-tooth comb   H. used to remove excess or unwanted hair at the neckline and
                                            around ears
    _____ 9. sectioning clips   I. used to detangle hair

44. Why is the way you hold your tools so important?

   a) _____

   b) _____

45. Describe the proper way to hold shears.

   _____

   _____

46. Which hand will be your cutting hand and what will it do?

   _____

   _____

47. Which hand is your holding hand and what does it do?

   _____

   _____

48. Identify what is happening in each of the following illustrations

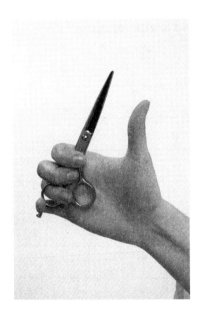

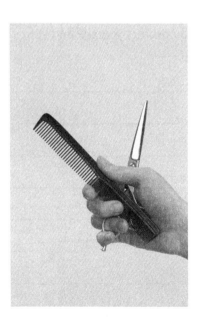

   _____   _____

49. What is the straight razor or shaping razor used for?

   _____

50. _____ in haircutting is the amount of pressure applied when combing and holding a subsection, created by stretching or pulling the subsection.

51. What steps can you take to insure that you are using good posture and body position when cutting hair?

    a) _____

    _____

    b) _____

    _____

    c) _____

    _____

52. Match the following hand positions to the cut they deliver.

    _____ 1. over fingers   A. used to cut a one-length bob or a heavier graduated haircut

    _____ 2. below fingers   B. used to maintain control of the subsection, with regard to elevation and overdirection

    _____ 3. palm-to-palm   C. used when cutting uniform or increasing layers

53. How can you protect yourself and your client from the sharp blades and instruments used in haircutting?

    a) _____

    _____

    b) _____

    _____

    c) _____

    _____

    d) _____

    _____

    e) _____

    _____

    f) _____

    _____

54. To maintain the proper sanitation of your station and supplies you must do the following for each client.

a) _____

_____

b) _____

_____

c) _____

_____

d) _____

_____

e) _____

_____

f) _____

_____

g) _____

_____

BASIC HAIRCUTS

55. Which of the following haircuts is not one of the four basic haircuts that all haircutting stems from?

_____ a) blunt cut

_____ b) graduated cut

_____ c) wedge cut

_____ d) layered cut

56. In a _____ all the hair comes to one hanging level, forming a weight line or area.

57. What is a weight line?

_____

58. What's another name for a blunt cut?

_____a)   a 45-degree elevation cut

_____b)   a 90-degree elevation cut

_____c)   a zero-elevation cut

_____d)   a 120-degree elevation cut

59. Blunt haircuts are particularly suitable for:

_____a)   thick hair

_____b)   coarse hair

_____c)   thin hair

_____d)   medium coarse hair

60. A _____ is a graduated shape or wedge, an effect or haircut that results from

cutting the hair with tension, low to medium elevation, or overdirection.

61. The most commonly used elevations are 45 degrees and:

_____a)   180

_____b)   30

_____c)   90

_____d)   60

62. In a graduated haircut there is a visual buildup of _____ in a given area.

a) tension

b) weight

c) syling product

d) color

63. A _____ is a graduated effect achieved by cutting the hair with elevation or

overdirection.

64. Layers create _____ and _____ in the hair by releasing weight.

65. The _____ is cut at a 180-degree angle, which gives more volume to the hairstyle

and can be combined with other basic haircuts.

66. The shape of a long layered haircut is

_____ .

67. What position should the client's head be in when cutting a blunt cut?

_____

68. List the implements and materials you will need to cut a blunt cut.

a) _____   f) _____

b) _____   g) _____

c) _____   h) _____

d) _____   i) _____

e) _____

69. Describe what is happening in the illustrations below.

_____

_____

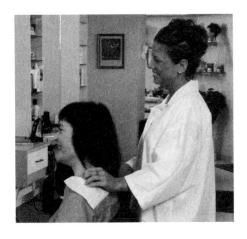 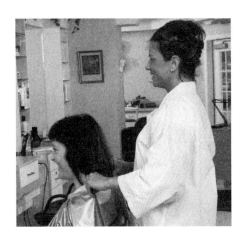

70. How should the hair be parted when cutting a blunt cut?

_____

71. For a blunt cut, how many sections should you part the hair into and where are the sections?

_____

_____

72. How should you begin the haircut?

_____

73. How should you create your guideline for this cut?

_____

_____

_____

74. How should you continue to cut the back?

_____

75. How should you match the sides of the haircut to the back?

_____

_____

_____

76. Once the cut is completed, how will you cross-check the haircut?

_____

_____

77. Once the haircut is dry, how will you best check the cut?

_____

_____

78. For the _____ you will be working with a vertical cutting line and a 45-degree

and a 90-degree elevation.

79. Before you begin to cut a graduated haircut, how many sections should the hair be divided into?

_____ a) two

_____ b) four

_____ c) five

_____ d) six

80. To establish your guideline you will first cut _____ .

81. Describe the action taking place in this illustration.

_____

_____

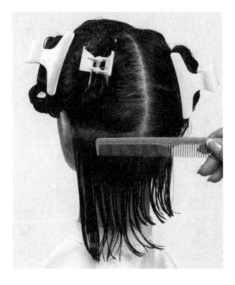

82. Once you extend the subsection from the top down to include the nape guideline, you will comb the subsection smooth at a 45-degree angle to the scalp and you will hold your fingers at a _____ angle to the strand to cut.

83. As you continue to cut the hair it will gradually become _____ as it reaches the apex.

84. What is happening in this illustration?

_____

_____

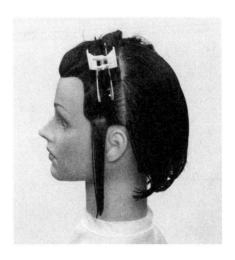

85. How should you blend the hair in the left side section with those in the upper crown area?

_____

_____

86. What action is being taken in this illustration?

_____

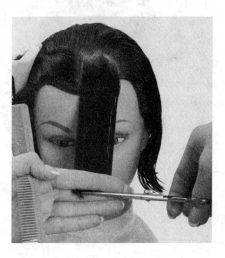

87. How will you finish the top of the haircut?

_____

_____

88. Name two other graduated haircuts.

_____

89. When working with coarse textures and curly hair you should keep your elevation below _____

to avoid excessive graduation.

90. Why does fine hair respond well to graduation?

_____

91. The basic layered haircut is created with _____ .

92. With a uniform layered cut, all the hair is elevated to _____ degrees and cut at the same length.

93. What is an interior guideline?

_____

94. What effect does a layered haircut have on weight lines?

_____ a)   builds up weight lines

_____ b)   decreases weight lines

_____ c)   eliminates all weight lines

95. To create the guideline for a layered cut you should take two partings ½ inch apart, creating a section

that runs from the _____ to the _____.

96. Describe what is occurring in these illustrations.

_____

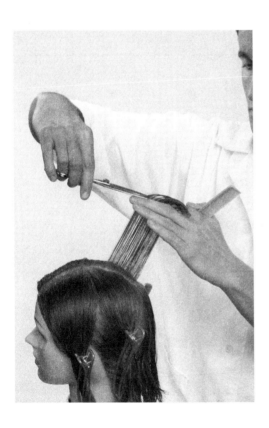
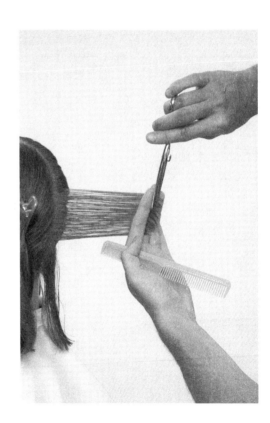

97. How can you maintain control and consistency while working through the layered haircut?

_____

98. When you begin to cut the interior hair in a layered haircut, you should _____

_____ .

99. When you begin cutting on the left side, shift your body position so that the tips of your shears are

pointing _____ and the fingers holding the section are pointing _____ .

100. How should you cross-check the entire back area?

_____

101. What is being pictured here?

_____

_____

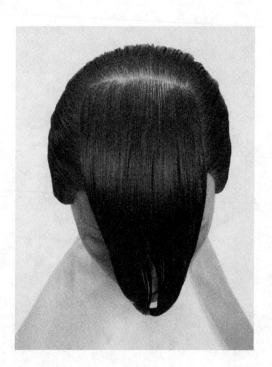

102. When cutting the top area you should use_____ partings and be careful not to

_____ the hair so that the layers remain a uniform length.

103. When cutting the sides you should work from the _____ ,

    using vertical sections.

    a) front of the face to the back of the ear

    b) back of the ear to the front of the face

104. How is a long layered haircut achieved?

    _____

    _____

105. For a long layered haircut, how many sections will you part the hair into?

    _____ a) three

    _____ b) four

    _____ c) five

    _____ d) six

106. List the steps involved in completing a long layered haircut

    a) _____

    _____

    b) _____

    _____

    c) _____

    _____

    d) _____

    _____

    e) _____

    _____

    f) _____

    _____

    g) _____

    _____

    h) _____

    _____

CUTTING CURLY HAIR

107. What is the most important thing to remember when cutting curly hair?

_____

108. Curly hair _____ much more after it dries than straight hair.

    a) extends

    b) changes color

    c) shrinks

    d) straightens

109. Match the illustration below to the term that best describes it.

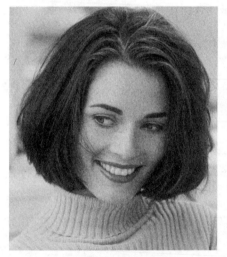 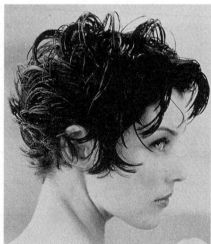 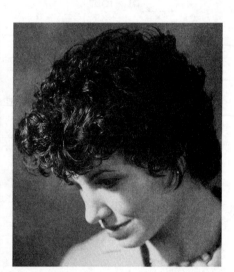

_____   _____   _____

_____   _____   _____

OTHER CUTTING TECHNIQUES

110. Where is the fringe area of a haircut?

_____

_____

111. Does the hair in the fringe area always have to be blended with the rest of the haircut? What is the determining factor?

_____

112. What kind of effect is achieved with a razor cut?

_____

113. When using a razor, where will the guide be?

_____

114. Are there any hair types or conditions that you should not use a razor on?

_____

115. Why should you always use a new, sharp blade when razor cutting?

_____

116. When using a razor you may cut the hair either wet or dry.

_____ True

_____ False

117. _____ is a method of cutting or thinning the hair in which the fingers and

shears glide along the edge of the hair to remove length.

118. Slide cutting is useful for:

a) _____

b) _____

c) _____

119. How is slide cutting accomplished?

_____

120. _____ is a technique in which you hold the hair in place with the comb while

you use the tips of the shears to remove the lengths.

121. List the basic steps in working with the shears over-comb technique.

a) _____

b) _____

_____

c) _____

_____

d) _____

_____

122. _____ is the process of removing excess bulk without shortening the length

and cutting for effect within the hair length, causing wispy or spiky effects.

123. What are texturizing techniques used for within a haircut?

a) _____

b) _____

c) _____

d) _____

124. What tools are used for texturizing?

_____

125. Match each of the following texturizing techniques with the phrase that best describes it

_____ 1. point-cutting   A.   used to remove bulk and add movement through the lengths of
                                      the hair

_____ 2. notching   B.   used on the interior of cut to release curl and remove density

_____ 3. free-hand notching   C.   creates a visual separation in the hair

_____ 4. slithering   D.   a technique performed on hair ends to cut points in the hair

_____ 5. slicing   E.   creates texture and separation at the perimeter of a haircut

_____ 6. carving   F.   thinning the hair to graduated lengths with shears

_____ 7. carving the ends   G.   an aggressive form of point-cutting, creating a chunkier effect

126. Thinning shears were originally created for the purpose of _____ and

_____.

127. List the ways that a thinning shears can be used to remove weight from a haircut.

a) _____

b) _____

128. Can a razor be used to accomplish texturizing? If so, using what techniques?

_____

_____

129. What is the razor rotation technique used for?

_____

CLIPPERS, EDGERS, AND TRIMMERS

130. What are clippers?

_____

_____

131. List all the tools to have on hand when clipper cutting

a) _____

b) _____

c) _____

d) _____

e) _____

f) _____

132. The clipper-over-comb technique allows you to

_____

133. List the implements and materials needed to complete a clipper cut.

a) _____

b) _____

c) _____

d) _____

e) _____

f) _____

g) _____

h) _____

134. How should you part the hair for a clipper cut?

_____

_____

135. Where and how should you begin the clipper cut?

_____

_____

_____

136. How do you blend the sections with the clipper?

_____

137. To cut the hair very close from the sideburn to the parietal ridge you should use a

_____ .

138. How should you determine the guideline for the length in the crown area?

_____

_____

139. When working with clippers you should always work _____ the natural growth patterns,

especially in the nape.

a) with

b) against

140. When using the clipper-over-comb technique, try to cut all the way across the entire length of the comb.

_____ True

_____ False

141. When using the clipper-over-comb technique, the angle of the comb determines the cutting angle.

    _____ True

    _____ False

142. Edgers, also called _____ , are usually smaller-sized clippers.

143. Where are edgers most commonly used?

    _____

144. Can clippers and edgers be used to trim beards and mustaches?

    _____

145. How should you use a clipper to remove length from a beard?

    _____

12

HAIRSTYLING

Date: _____

Rating _____

Text Pages: 347-421

POINT TO PONDER:

"Citizens may be born free; they are not born wise. Therefore the business of liberal education in a democracy is to make free men wise."—F Champion Ward

1. Determining the perfect hairstyling technique to use for a client is dependant on his or her _____ _____ and _____ and your practical skill level.

CLIENT CONSULTATION

2. What is the best way for a client to convey her expectations to you in terms of what she prefers in a hair-style?

_____

3. What factors will help you and the client make a final decision on an appropriate design?

_____

WET HAIRSTYLING BASICS

4. List the most commonly used wet hairstyling tools.

a) _____   d) _____

b) _____   e) _____

c) _____   f) _____

5. List the implements and materials you will need to prepare for wet hairstyling.

a) _____   c) _____

b) _____   d) _____

6. How will you prepare yourself and your client for wet hairstyling?

   a) _____

   b) _____

   c) _____

   d) _____

   e) _____

7. Describe what action is taking place in the illustrations below.

   _____

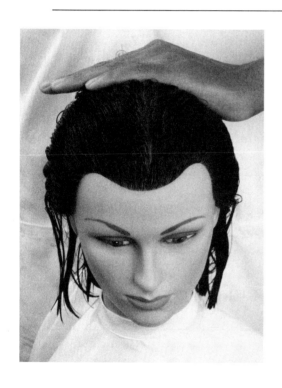 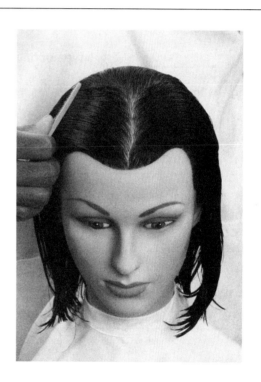

8. What is a natural part?

   _____

9. How can you determine the client's natural part?

   a) _____

   b) _____

   c) _____

FINGER WAVING

10. Finger waving is the process of _____

    through the use of the fingers, combs, and waving lotion.

11. Why should you bother to learn finger waving now, since it hasn't been in style since the 1920s and 1930s?

    _____

    _____

    _____

12. _____ is a type of hair gel that makes the hair pliable enough to keep it in

    place during the finger waving procedure.

13. How will you know if you have used too much waving lotion on the hair?

    _____

14. What side of the head should a finger wave be started on? The left or right?

    _____

15. What is the special term used to indicate the side where the wave is usually started?

    _____

16. List all of the implements and materials required for finger waving

    a) _____   d) _____

    b) _____   e) _____

    c) _____

17. After shampooing and before applying waving lotion you should: _____

    _____.

18. How should you apply waving lotion?

    _____

    _____

19. To begin the first wave on the right side of the head, using the index finger of your _____

    _____ hand as a guide, shape the top hair with a comb into the beginning of the

    _____ shaping, using a circular movement.

20. You should begin at the:

    _____ a) forehead
    _____ b) hairline
    _____ c) nape
    _____ d) ear

21. When forming the first ridge, what position should the teeth of the comb be pointing in?

    _____

    _____

    _____

22. To form the second ridge, begin at the _____ area.

23. The movements are the same as those followed in forming the first ridge.

    _____ True

    _____ False

24. Both the ridge and the wave must blend, without _____, with the ridge and wave on

    the right side of the head.

25. Once the entire head is finger waved, what should you do?

    _____

    _____

    _____

26. Once dry, remove the client from under the dryer and let the hair _____ before

    removing all clips or pins and the hairnet from the hair.

27. How should you finish off the style?

    _____

28. How should you clean up after this service?

_____

_____

29. Describe an alternate method of finger waving.

_____

_____

PIN CURLS

30. Pin curls serve as the basis for only one type of hairstyle.

_____ True

_____ False

31. Pin curls may be used only on hair that has been permanently waved.

_____ True

_____ False

32. Pin curls work best when the hair is properly layered and is smoothly wound.

_____ True

_____ False

33. Pin curls are made up of three principal parts _____.

34. The _____ is the stationary, or nonmoving, foundation of the curl, which is the area closest to the scalp.

35. The _____ is the section of the pin curl, between the base and first arc (turn) of the circle, that gives the circle its direction and movement.

36. The _____ is the part of the pin curl that forms a complete circle. Its size determines the width of the wave and its strength.

37. Label the three parts of the pin curl on this illustration

    a) _____

    b) _____

    c) _____

38. The _____ determines the amount of mobility, or movement, of a section of hair.

    a) base

    b) stem

    c) circle

39. Curl mobility is classified as

    a) _____

    b) _____

    c) _____

40. The _____ curl is placed directly on the base of the curl, produces a tight, firm, long-lasting curl, and allows minimum mobility.

41. The _____ curl permits medium movement; the curl is placed half off the base and it gives good control to the hair.

42. The _____ curl allows for the greatest mobility because the curl is placed completely off the base and gives as much freedom as the length of the stem will permit.

43. The base of a full-stem curl may be what shape?

    _____

    _____

44. A _____ is a section of hair that is molded in a circular movement in preparation for the formation of curls.

45. Shapings are either _____ or _____ .

46. Where should you always begin a pin curl?

    _____

47. _____ curls produce even, smooth waves and uniform curls.

48. _____ curls produce waves that get smaller in size toward the end.

49. When would you use the closed center curl?

_____

50. Label the center curls illustrated below.

_____   _____

51. What is a clockwise curl?

_____

52. What is a counterclockwise curl?

_____

53. The most commonly used pin curl bases are

a) _____   c) _____

b) _____   d) _____

54. To avoid splits in the finished hairstyle, you must use care when _____

_____.

55. Where are rectangular base pin curls used?

_____

56. Where are triangular base pin curls used?

_____

57. Where are arc base pin curls used?

_____

58. When are square base pin curls used?

_____

59. To avoid splits when combing out a pin curl set, you should _____ the sectioning.

60. The technique which involves forcing the hair between the thumb and the back of the comb to create tension is called:

_____ a) threading
_____ b) ribboning
_____ c) slicing
_____ d) sculpting

61. Pin curls sliced from a shaping and formed without lifting the hair from the head are referred to as

_____.

62. List the implements and materials you will need for pin curling

a) _____
b) _____
c) _____

63. Describe the procedure for making a pin curl:

a) _____
b) _____
c) _____
d) _____
e) _____

64. Describe the correct and incorrect placing of the clip illustrated below,

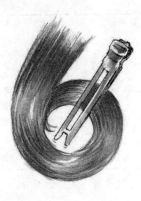 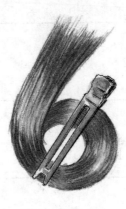

_____   _____

_____   _____

_____   _____

65. How can you use pin curls to create a wave?

_____

66. How are pin curls used to create ridge curls?

_____

67. What are skip waves?

_____

_____

68. Cascade or stand-up curls are used to create _____ in the hair design.

69. What position are cascade curls fastened in?

_____

_____

70. What are barrel curls?

_____

_____

71. What effect can you get from a barrel curl?

_____

ROLLER CURLS

72. What are the advantages of using rollers over pin curls?

a) _____

_____

b) _____

_____

c) _____

_____

73. Identify the three parts of the roller curl, using this illustration.

1. _____

2. _____

3. _____

74. What is the base?

_____

75. How big should the base be?

_____

76. What is the stem?

_____

77. What is the function of the stem?

_____

78. What is the curl or circle?

_____

79. Why is the size of the circle important?

_____

80. Match the following type of curl with the description of how it is wound.

    _____   1.   one complete turn around the roller   A. curls

    _____   2.   one and a half turns around the roller   B. c-shaped curl

    _____   3.   two and a half turns around the roller   C. wave

81. The _____ of the roller and how it sits on its _____ will determine the volume you

can achieve from a roller set.

82. What type of volume will you get from an on-base curl?

_____

83. What type of volume will you get from a half base curl?

_____

84. What type of volume will you get from an off-base curl?

_____

85. List the implements and materials needed for a wet set with rollers.

   a) _____   c) _____

   b) _____   d) _____

86. To begin the wet set you should _____

_____.

87. Begin setting the rollers at the _____ , and part off a section the same length and

width as the roller.

88. How will you determine what type of base to use?

_____

89. How smooth should the hair be before winding it around the roller?

_____

90. Hold the hair with tension between your thumb and middle finger and wrap the ends of the hair smoothly around the roller until the hair catches and does not release.

_____ True

_____ False

91. Use your _____ over the ends of the roller and roll the hair firmly to the scalp.

   a) combs

   b) brushes

   c) thumbs

   d) pinkies

92. How do you secure the roller to the scalp hair?

_____

93. Once the hair is dry, when should you remove the rollers?

_____

94. _____ rollers and _____ rollers are used on dry hair only.

95. How do hot rollers work?

_____

96. How long should hot rollers be allowed to stay on the hair?

_____

97. What are Velcro rollers and how are they used?

_____

98. What type of client is best suited for a Velcro set?

_____

_____

99. How long do Velcro rollers stay in the hair?

_____

COMB-OUT TECHNIQUES

100. Following a well-structured system of combing out hairstyles allows you to: _____

_____ .

101. List the implements and materials you will need for combing out a wet set:

a) _____   c) _____

b) _____   d) _____

102. How should you drape a client for a comb-out?

_____

_____

103. After removing the rollers and clips, brush the hair through to _____ the set.

104. Smooth the hair and brush it into a high volume condition that permits you to position the lines for the planned hairstyle.

_____ True

_____ False

105. When combing out a curly style, use a _____ to lift and separate the curls before brushing

out the hair.

106. After brushing the hair, lines of direction should be slightly _____ to allow for

some relaxation during the comb-out process.

107. Areas that require volume should be _____ , and areas that need to be brought into

the set should be _____ .

108. You should attempt to comb and brush the entire style into place at one time.

_____ True

_____ False

109. After completing the comb-out, you can use the tail of a comb to _____

_____ .

110. When should you use a finishing spray?

_____

111. List the steps involved in cleaning up after a comb-out.

a) _____

b) _____

c) _____

d) _____

e) _____

112. List all of the alternative names for back-combing

a) _____ c) _____

b) _____ d) _____

113 What action is involved in back-combing?

_____

_____

114. What is back-brushing or ruffing?

_____

_____

115. What are back-combing and back-brushing mainly used for?

_____

_____

116. List the steps of the procedure for back-combing.

a) _____

_____

b) _____

_____

c) _____

_____

d) _____

_____

117. Give the procedure for back-brushing.

a) _____

b) _____

_____

_____

c) _____

d) _____

_____

HAIR WRAPPING

118. If you are working with curly hair, the technique known as _____ is sufficient

for a smooth, straight look.

119. What is the technique of wrapping hair used for?

_____

120. How is wrapping done?

_____

_____

121. Wrapping can be done on wet hair only.

_____ True

_____ False

122. If you are working with very curly hair, you must first _____ and then wrap it.

123. List the implements and materials you will need for wrapping the hair.

a) _____   c) _____

b) _____

124. When should you use a gel or a silicone shine product?

_____

125. Where should your hand rest to hold the head during the wrap procedure?

_____

126. How will you wrap the hair around the head?

_____

_____

127. What will you use to keep the hair in place while wrapping?

_____

128. What should your free hand be doing while you continue wrapping the hair in a clockwise direction around the head?

_____

129. Once all the hair is wrapped you should: _____

_____

130. If working on dry hair, leave the hair wrapped for about _____ minutes.

    a) five

    b) 15

    c) 30

    d) 45

131. If working on wet hair, place the client under a hooded dryer until the hair is completely dry, usually _____ minutes, depending on the hair length.

    a) five

    b) 15

    c) 30

    d) 45

BLOW-DRY STYLING

132. Blow-dry styling is the technique of _____ damp hair in one operation.

133. A _____ is an electrical device designed for drying and styling hair in a single service.

134. Name the main parts of the blow-dryer.

    a) _____   d) _____

    b) _____   e) _____

    c) _____

135. The blow-dryer's nozzle attachment, or _____ , is a directional feature that directs

    the air stream to any section of the hair more intensely.

136. The _____ attachment causes the air to flow more softly and helps to accentuate or

    keep textural definition.

137. What can happen if your blow-dryer is unclean?

    _____

138. Combs and picks are designed to _____ and _____ the hair.

139. Combs with teeth that are closely spaced _____ definition from the curl, thus creating a

    smooth surface.

140. Combs with wide spaces between teeth _____ larger sections of hair for more surface

    texture.

141. Combs with picks at one end serve to _____ .

142. Describe a classic styling brush.

    _____

    _____

143. What are classic styling brushes best used for?

_____

_____

144. Describe a paddle brush and what it is used for.

_____

_____

145. _____ are oval with pure natural bristles or quills of bristle-and-nylon mix.

146. Grooming brushes with _____ bristles help distribute the scalp oils throughout the shaft of

the hair, giving it shine, while the _____ ____bristles stimulate the circulation of blood to the scalp.

147. For what purpose are grooming brushes best used?

_____

148. _____ brushes, with their ventilated design, are used to speed up the blow-drying

process, and are ideal for blow-drying fine hair and adding lift at the scalp.

149. How are round brushes used?

_____

_____

150. Why do some round brushes have metal cylinder bases?

_____

_____

151. A _____ is a nylon styling brush that has a tail for sectioning, along with a

narrow row of bristles.

152. Teasing brushes are used for _____

_____.

153. _____ clips are usually metal or plastic and have long prongs to hold wet or dry

sections of hair in place.

154. Styling lotions can be thought of as _____.

155. What questions must you answer before choosing the right styling aid to use?

a) _____

b) _____

c) _____

d) _____

156. Foam or mousse builds _____body and volume into the hair.

157. How is mousse used?

_____

_____

158. What hair texture is best served with a foam product?

_____

159. When is gel used?

_____

_____

160. When are liquid gels or texturizers used?

_____

161. How are straightening gels used?

_____

_____

162. When sprayed into the base of fine, wet hair,_____ add volume to the shape,

especially at the base, when the hair is blown dry.

163. How is pomade, or wax, used?

_____

_____

164. _____ add gloss and sheen to the hair while creating textural definition.

165. _____ , or finishing spray, is the most widely used hairstyling product and is

effective to hold the style in place.

166. What is a working spray?

_____

167. List all of the implements and materials needed for blow-dry styling.

a) _____   d) _____

b) _____   e) _____

c) _____   f) _____

168. How should you prepare for blow-dry styling?

a) _____

b) _____

c) _____

169. List the steps you should follow to blow-dry short, layered, curly hair to get a smooth and full finish.

a) _____

b) _____

c) _____

_____

d) _____

e) _____

f) _____

_____

g) _____

170. List the steps you should follow to blow-dry short, curly hair in its natural wave pattern.

a) _____

b) _____

c) _____

d) _____

_____

e) _____

_____

f) _____

171. List the steps you should follow to diffuse long, curly or extremely curly hair in its natural wave pattern,

a) _____

b) _____

c) _____

_____

d) _____

172. List the steps you should follow to blow-dry straight or wavy hair with maximum volume.

a) _____

b) _____

c) _____

d) _____

e) _____

_____

f) _____

g) _____

_____

h) _____

i) _____

173. List the steps you should follow to blow-dry blunt or long layered, straight to wavy hair into a smooth straight style.

a) _____

b) _____

c) _____

d) _____

_____

e) _____

f) _____

_____

g) _____

h) _____

i) _____

j) _____

k) _____

l) _____

174. Describe the cleanup and sanitation steps you should follow when the blow dry is completed.

a) _____

b) _____

c) _____

d) _____

e) _____

STYLING LONG HAIR

175. Describe an updo.

_____

_____

176. Describe a chignon.

_____

177. List all of the implements and materials you will need to style a chignon.

a) _____   f) _____

b) _____   g) _____

c) _____   h) _____

d) _____   i) _____

e) _____   j) _____

178. How will you prepare your client for styling a chignon?

a) _____

b) _____

c) _____

d) _____

e) _____

179. Using a _____

_____ .

180. How should you secure the ponytail?

_____

181. How will you conceal the elastic band?

_____

_____

182. Once the elastic is concealed, smooth out the ponytail and begin _____ from

underneath the ponytail.

183. How is the chignon formed?

_____

184. How should you secure the underside of the roll?

_____

185. How do you conceal the bobby pins?

   _____

186. Finish the style with a light working spray.

   _____ True

   _____ False

187. If you want to add flowers or ornaments to the style when is that done?

   _____

188. List the steps in the procedure for a basic French twist:

   a) _____

   b) _____

   _____

   c) _____

   _____

   d) _____

189. How is a classic French twist different from a basic French twist?

   _____

190. To start, you should section off the _____ area and the two side sections.

191. How is the back area prepared for the classic French twist?

   _____

192. Where do you begin pinning the hair?

   _____

   _____

193. How do you conceal the bobby pins you just secured?

   _____

   _____

194. How do you secure this hair?

_____

195. What should you do with the hair ends?

_____

196. How should you style the side sections?

_____

_____

197. List the steps required for styling the top section.

a) _____

b) _____

_____

c) _____

_____

d) _____

e) _____

f) _____

_____

198. How should you finish the side area?

_____

199. How should you style the bangs?

_____

_____

200. How should you finish off the twist?

_____

THERMAL HAIRSTYLING

201. What is thermal waving and thermal curling?

   _____

   _____

202. Thermal irons provide an _____ and are made of the best quality _____

   so that they hold an even temperature during the waving and curling process.

203. The styling portion of the irons is composed of two parts, the _____ and the _____ .

204. The edge of the shell nearest the stylist is called the _____ and the one farthest from the

   stylist is called the _____ .

205. Name the three different classifications of thermal irons.

   a) _____   c) _____

   b) _____

206. How do you determine the correct temperature for thermal styling?

   _____

   _____

207. What is the best way to test an iron's temperature?

   _____

   _____

208. How should you remove dirt or grease from a thermal iron?

   _____

   _____

209. How long should the comb be that you use with a thermal iron?

   _____ a)   about 3" long
   _____ b)   about 5" long
   _____ c)   about 7" long
   _____ d)   about 9" long

210. What should the comb be made of?

_____ a) hard plastic

_____ b) soft plastic

_____ c) hard rubber

_____ d) soft plastic

211. What is the best way to practice holding and manipulating the thermal irons?

_____

_____

212. List the implements and materials you will need for thermal waving with conventional thermal irons.

a) _____   d) _____

b) _____   e) _____

c) _____

213. What steps should you take to prepare your client for the procedure?

a) _____

b) _____

c) _____

214. What is the deciding factor for whether or not the first wave will be a left-going wave or a right-going wave?

_____

215. The first step is to _____ the hair thoroughly, following its directional growth.

a) brush

b   comb

c) tease

d) cut

216. How much hair should you pick up to curl at one time?

_____

217. Where should the groove of the iron be when you insert it into the hair?

_____

218. Once the iron is in the hair what should you do?

_____

_____

219. What is happening in the illustration below and why?

_____

220. How do you reverse the movement?

_____

221. How do you then place the iron below the ridge or crest you just made?

_____

_____

222. To form the hair into a half circle you need to _____

_____.

223. The second ridge is the beginning of a right-going wave, in which the hair is directed _____

to that of a left-going wave.

224. How should you clean up after the thermal waving procedure?

a) _____

b) _____

c) _____

d) _____

225. How is thermal curling used on a client with straight hair?

_____

_____

226. Can thermal curling used on a client with pressed hair?

_____

_____

227. Can thermal curling used on wigs and hairpieces?

_____

228. What method of holding the irons should you use?

_____

_____

229. Developing a smooth _____ movement is important in thermal curling, so practice

by turning the irons while opening and closing them at regular intervals.

230. How can you practice releasing the hair from the iron?

_____

231. Why should you practice guiding the hair strand into the center of the curl as you rotate the irons?

_____

232. How can you protect the client's scalp from burns while removing the curl from the irons?

_____

_____

233. How do you prepare your client for curling with thermal irons?

    a) _____

    b) _____

    c) _____

    d) _____

    e) _____

234. When curling short hair, where do you begin to curl?

    _____

    _____

235. The curl base is usually about 1-$\frac{1}{2}$" to 2" in width.

    _____ True

    _____ False

236. How deep should the base of the curl be?

    _____ $\frac{1}{4}$"
    _____ $\frac{1}{2}$"
    _____ $\frac{3}{4}$"
    _____   1"

237. After sectioning off the base, you should:

    _____ a)   wrap it around the iron
    _____ b)   wrap it around a roller
    _____ c)   comb the hair smooth and straight out from the scalp
    _____ d)   comb it down and flat against the scalp

238. Once the irons have been heated and you pick up a strand of hair and comb it up smoothly, insert the

    irons about _____ from the scalp and hold for a few seconds to form a base.

    a) $\frac{1}{4}$"
    b) $1\frac{1}{2}$"
    c) 1"
    d) 1-$\frac{1}{2}$"

239. How do you guide the rest of the hair strand into the iron for curling?

_____

_____

240. If you complete this successfully, what is the result of this procedure?

_____

241. When curling medium-length hair you will need to first _____.

242. To make the curl, you insert the hair into the open irons at the _____.

    a) midshaft

    b) scalp

    c) ends

    d) stem of the curl

243. Once the irons are in position, hold them for about _____ to heat the hair, and then

    slide the irons up to 1" from the scalp.

    a) five seconds

    b) 15 seconds

    c) 30 seconds

    d) one minute

244. Next, you turn the irons _____ one-half revolution

    a) upward

    b) to the left

    c) to the right

    d) downward

245. What is taking place in this illustration?

_____

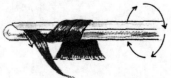

246. How do the ends become curled?

_____

_____

247. How can you smooth the ends and loosen the hair away from the irons?

_____

_____

248. To curl long hair you use two loops or _____ .

249. Start by _____ and _____ the base of the curl.

250. Insert the hair into the open irons about _____ from the scalp.

   a) ¼"

   b) ½"

   c) 1"

   d) 2"

251. In which direction should you pull the hair over the rod?

_____

252. How long should you hold the irons in this position?

_____

253. How much tension should you use when holding the strand of hair?

   _____ a)   no tension
   _____ b)   small amount of tension
   _____ c)   medium degree of tension
   _____ d)   great degree of tension

254. In what direction should you roll the irons?

   _____ a)   over
   _____ b)   under
   _____ c)   left
   _____ d)   right

255. How will you curl the rest if the strand?

_____

_____

_____

256. What will this pushing action accomplish?

_____

_____

257. How will you curl the ends?

_____

258. How can you be sure to even out the distribution of the hair in the curl and to facilitate the movement of the curl off the irons?

_____

259. What is a spiral curl?

_____

260. What kind of a look do spiral curls result in?

_____

261. How is a spiral curl created?

_____

_____

_____

_____

262. What are end curls?

_____

263. With end curls the hair ends are curled in what direction?

_____

264. _____ thermal iron curls are used to create volume or lift in a finished hairstyle.

265. What determines the type of volume curls to be used?

_____

266. Match the type of base curl with the volume it provides.

    _____ 1. volume-base curls   A. moderate volume

    _____ 2. full-base curls   B. slight volume

    _____ 3. half-base curls   C. maximum volume

    _____ 4. off-base curls   D. full volume

267. Why do volume-base curls provide maximum lift or volume?

_____

268. How is a volume-based curl wound?

_____

_____

_____

269. How is the curl placed on its base?

_____

270. How are full-base curls wound?

_____

_____

_____

271. What kind of a curl can you expect to get with a half-base curl?

_____

272. How is a half-base curl wound?

_____

_____

273. How is an off-base curl wound?

_____

_____

274. After the curls are made, how should they be fastened until you are ready to comb out the style?

_____

THERMAL HAIR STRAIGHTENING (HAIR PRESSING)

275. _____ temporarily straightens extremely curly or unruly hair by means of a

heated iron or comb.

276. How long does a pressing last?

_____

277. What additional services can hair pressing prepare the hair for?

_____

278. In what kind of condition does a good hair pressing leave the hair?

_____

279. Match the type of pressing with how much curl it removes from the hair.

_____ 1. soft press   A. removes about 60% to 75% of curl
_____ 2. medium press   B. removes 100% of curl
_____ 3. hard press   C. removes about 50% to 60% of curl

280. A soft press is accomplished by applying the thermal pressing comb _____ .

281. A medium press is accomplished by applying the thermal pressing comb _____

_____ .

282. A hard press involves applying the thermal pressing comb _____ on each side of the hair.

283. A hard press that is done by first passing a hot curling iron through the hair is called a _____ .

284. Before you press a client's hair, you need to analyze the condition of the _____ and _____ .

285. If you notice that the client's hair and scalp are not normal, what should you do?

_____

286. If the client's hair shows signs of neglect or abuse caused by faulty pressing, lightening, or tinting, what can you recommend?

_____

287. What can happen if you press hair that is dry and brittle?

_____

288. What two things do you need to check before agreeing to give a pressing?

_____

289. A careful analysis of the client's hair should cover the following points.

a) _____   e) _____

b) _____   f) _____

c) _____   g) _____

d) _____   h) _____

290. Why is it important to be able to recognize individual differences in hair texture, porosity, elasticity, and scalp flexibility?

_____

_____

291. Variations in hair texture have to do with the _____ of the hair and the _____ of the hair.

292. Coarse, extremely curly hair requires less heat and pressure than medium or fine hair in the pressing process.

_____ True

_____ False

293. Medium curly hair is the most resistant to hair pressing.

_____ True

_____ False

294. To avoid hair breakage of fine hair, less heat and pressure should be applied than for other hair textures.

_____ True

_____ False

295. What are the two layers found in fine hair?

_____

296. What does wiry, curly hair feel like?

_____

297. What makes wiry hair resistant to hair pressing?

_____

298. Does wiry hair require more or less heat and pressure than other types of hair?

_____

299. What are the three classifications of a client's scalp condition?

_____

300. If the scalp is tight and the hair coarse, how should you press the hair?

_____

301. What is the main difficulty with a flexible scalp?

_____

302. Should you keep a record card for pressing services?

_____

_____

303. When should you ask the client about any lightener, tint, color restorer, or other chemical treatment that has been used on the hair?

_____

304. Does the application of a conditioning treatment usually enhance or detract from the results of hair pressing?

_____

305. Can a tight scalp be made more flexible? How?

_____

306. What are the two types of pressing combs?

_____

307. What are pressing combs made of?

_____

308. A comb with more space between the teeth produces a _____ .

309. A comb with less space between the teeth produces a _____ press.

310. Pressing combs are all the same size.

_____ True

_____ False

311. Why should you temper a new pressing comb if it is made of brass?

_____

_____

312. If the polish is not burned off of a new pressing comb what can occur?

_____

313. How should you temper a new pressing comb?

_____

_____

_____

314. Name the two ways that pressing combs are heated.

_____

315. While the comb is being heated, its teeth should face _____ and the handle should be

kept away from the fire.

   a) downward

   b) upward

   c) to the left

   d) to the right

316. After heating the comb to the proper temperature, test it on _____.

317. How will you know if the comb is too hot?

_____

_____

318. Electric pressing combs are available in two forms. Describe them.

   a) _____

   b) _____

319. How should you clean the pressing comb?

_____

320. How can you remove the carbon from the comb?

_____

_____

_____

321. What are the reasons for using pressing oil or cream?

   a) _____

   b) _____

   c) _____

   d) _____

   e) _____

   f) _____

   g) _____

322. List all the implements and materials you need to do a soft press on normal curly hair.

a) _____   g) _____

b) _____   h) _____

c) _____   i) _____

d) _____   j) _____

e) _____   k) _____

f) _____   l) _____

323. After you have shampooed, rinsed, and towel-dried the client's hair, drape the client for thermal styling,

using a _____ and_____ .

324. When should you apply pressing oil or cream?

_____

325. How many sections should you divide the hair into for pressing?

_____

326. When should you place the pressing comb in the heater?

_____

327. Should you attempt to press one whole section at once?

_____

328. Before applying the pressing comb to the hair you should: _____

_____ .

329. How should you first insert the pressing comb?

_____

_____

330. How do you wrap the rest of the strand around the comb?

_____

_____

331. What part of the comb actually does the pressing?

_____

332. Where should you place each completed hair section?

_____

333. Once you have completed pressing all of the hair, what might you apply before brushing through the hair?

_____

334. Once the pressing is completed how should you finish the styling?

_____

335. List the cleanup and sanitation steps after pressing.

a) _____   d) _____

b) _____   e) _____

c) _____

336. When is a hard press recommended?

_____

337. How is a hard press completed?

_____

338. A hard press is also known as a _____.

339. What may cause pressed hair to become curly again?

_____

340. If the hair becomes curly again, what can be done about it?

_____

341. What two types of injuries can occur in hair pressing?

_____

_____

_____

342. To avoid damage and to ensure the client's safety avoid using the following.

a) _____

b) _____

c) _____

d) _____

343. When pressing fine hair be sure to not use a _____ pressing comb or too much _____ .

344. To avoid hair breakage during a pressing, apply less pressure to the hair near the _____ .

345. When pressing short, fine hair you must take extra care at the _____ .

    a) forehead

    b) nape

    c) ears

    d) hairline

346. When the hair is extra short, a pressing comb that is too hot will _____ .

347. If you burn the client's skin or scalp during a pressing service what should you do immediately?

_____

348. When pressing coarse hair be sure to apply enough pressure so that the hair remains _____ .

349. When pressing lightened or tinted hair the client may need _____

_____ .

350. Since gray hair may be resistant, use a _____ pressing comb applied with _____ pressure.

13

BRAIDING AND BRAID EXTENSIONS

Date: _____

Rating:_____

Text Pages: 423-455

POINT TO PONDER:

"It is the calling of great men, not so much to preach new truths, as to rescue from oblivion old truths it is our wisdom to remember and our weakness to forget."—Sidney Smith

1. The art of braiding has traditionally had social and cultural significance. Some examples are:

   a) _____

   b) _____

   c) _____

   _____

   d) _____

   _____

2. Braiding salons in many urban areas in the United States practice what is commonly known as

   _____.

CLIENT CONSULTATION

3. How long can it take to complete a complicated braided design?

   _____

4. Every braiding service should begin with a client consultation to prevent _____

   and to ensure _____ in the style.

5. During the consultation, when analyzing the condition of your client's hair, you must be particularly

   aware of the _____.

6. When discussing braiding and other natural hairstyling, texture refers to:

    a) _____   c) _____

    b) _____

7. The diameter of the hair indicates whether the hair is _____ , _____ , or _____ .

8. When determining the feel of the hair, you want to know if it feels:

    _____ .

9. When determining the hair's wave pattern you are discerning whether the hair is:

    _____ .

10. Describe coiled hair.

    _____

    _____

11. In addition to texture, what other characteristics should you observe about the hair?

    _____

12. If the hair at the hairline is weak or damaged you should avoid choosing certain braiding styles that place direct _____ on the hairline or partings along the hairline.

13. Match each of the following braiding styles with the face shape it is best suited for:

    _____ 1. oval face

    _____ 2. round face

    _____ 3. square face

    _____ 4. diamond face

    _____ 5. triangular face

    _____ 6. heart-shaped face

    _____ 7. oblong face

    A. updo or asymmetrical braiding styles that create the illusion of thinness

    B. soft bangs and wisps of curls along the face, avoid middle parts to create fullness around face

    C. braid styles that have soft fringes at the forehead and are close at the ears.

    D. full styles that create the illusion of length and to soften facial lines

    E. most braided styles are appropriate for this facial shape

    F. styles with full or partial bangs will fill-in around the forehead or jaw line

    G. full bang and full braids at chin will add fullness around the chin

UNDERSTANDING THE BASICS

14. What is the advantage of using a boar-bristle brush?

    _____

15. How do you use a square paddle brush?

    _____

    _____

16. What is the vent brush used for?

    _____

17. List all the tools you will need to complete a braiding service.

    a) _____   g) _____

    b) _____   h) _____

    c) _____   i) _____

    d) _____   j) _____

    e) _____   k) _____

    _____   l) _____

18. Extensions are most commonly made of:

    a) _____   e) _____

    b) _____   f) _____

    c) _____   g) _____

    d) _____

19. What is kanekalon and why is it a good choice for extensions?

    _____

    _____

    _____

    _____

20. Describe the pros and cons of nylon or rayon synthetic extensions.

_____

_____

_____

_____

21. Describe yarn and its use as a hair extension:

_____

_____

_____

_____

22. Describe lin and its use as a hair extension:

_____

_____

_____

23. Describe yak and its use as a hair extension.

_____

_____

24. Describe the use of a hackle in the hair extension process.

_____

_____

25. What is the drawing board and what is it used for?

_____

_____

_____

26. It is best to braid hair when it is dry.

_____ True

_____ False

27. List all the implements and materials needed for the braiding service.

a) _____   f) _____

b) _____   g) _____

c) _____   h) _____

d) _____   _____

e) _____

28. List the steps necessary to prepare for the braiding service.

a) _____

b) _____

c) _____

d) _____

e) _____

29. Describe the process for drying the hair before braiding.

a) _____

_____

b) _____

_____

c) _____

_____

d) _____

_____

e) _____

_____

f) _____

_____

g) _____

_____

h) _____

_____

_____

BRAIDING THE HAIR

30. What is a visible braid?

_____

_____

31. What is an invisible braid?

_____

_____

32. What implements and materials are needed to do an invisible braid?

a) _____   c) _____

b) _____   d) _____

33. Match the following descriptions with the photo that it describes to complete an invisible braid.

A. With your left hand, pick up a 1" section on the left side. Add this section to the left outer strand (1) in your right hand.

B. Move down the head with alternating pick-up movements and continue these movements until the braid is complete. Secure with a rubber band.

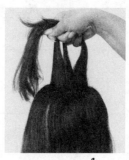
_____ 1.
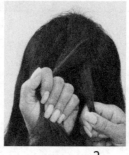
_____ 2.
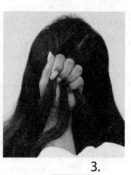
_____ 3.

C. Take the combined strands and cross them over the center strand.

D. Cross the left strand (3) over the center section and place it in your right hand. Place all three strands in your left hand with your fingers separating the strands.

E. Place all three sections in your left hand, pick up on the right side, and add to the outer strand (3).

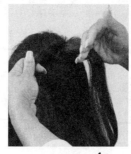
_____ 4.
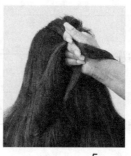
_____ 5.
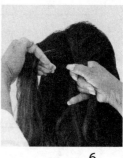
_____ 6.

F. At the crown of the head, take a triangular section of hair and place it in your left hand. Divide the section into three equal strands, two in your left hand, and one in your right.

G. Take the combined strands in your right hand and cross them over the center strand. Place all the strands in your right hand.

H. With your right hand, pick up a 1" section of hair on the right side. Add to strand (2) in your left hand.

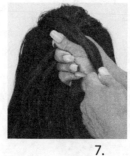
_____ 7.
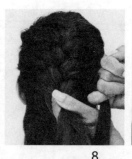
_____ 8.
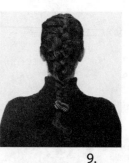
_____ 9.

I. Cross the right strand (1) over the center strand (2). Strand(1) is now the new center, and strand (2) is now on the right.

34. What is a rope braid?

35. Match the following descriptions with the photo that it describes to complete a rope braid.

A. With your hand in this position, twist toward the left (counter-clockwise) until your palm is facing down.

B. Cross the right strand over the left strand. Place both strands in your right hand with your index finger in between and your palm facing upward.

C. Twist the palm down (counter-clockwise), right strand over left.

D. Repeat, working toward the nape until the style is done. Secure with a rubber band.

E. Repeat these steps until you reach the end of the hair. Secure ends with a rubber band.

F. Pick up a 1" section from the left side. Add this section to the left strand.

G. When you run out of sections twist the left strand clockwise (to the right) two or three times. Place the strands in your right hand, index finger in between and palm up.

H. Put both strands in your left hand with the index finger in between and your palm up.

I. Divide the section into two equal strands.

J. Put both strands in your right hand with your index finger in between and your palm up.

K. Take a triangular section of hair from the front.

L. Pick up a 1" section from the right side and add it to the right strand.

M. Twist the left strand two times clockwise (toward the center).

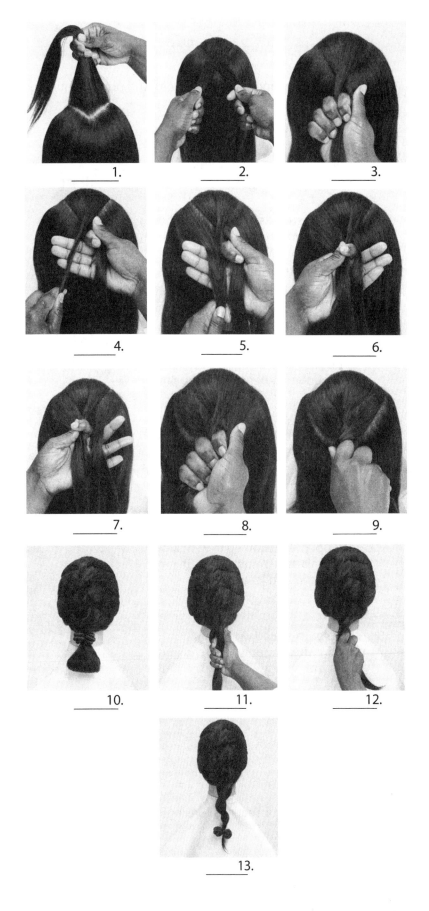

_____ 1.

_____ 2.

_____ 3.

_____ 4.

_____ 5.

_____ 6.

_____ 7.

_____ 8.

_____ 9.

_____ 10.

_____ 11.

_____ 12.

_____ 13.

36. What is a fishtail braid?

_____

_____

37. Match the following descriptions with the photo that it describes to complete a fishtail braid:

A. Pick up a 1" section on the right side. Cross this section over the right strand and add it to the left strand. You have now completed an X shape.

B. Put both strands in the right hand. Repeat steps moving your hand down toward the nape with each new section picked up.

C. Cross the right strand over the left strand.

D. Put both strands in the left hand, index finger in between and palm up.

E. Secure the hair with a rubber band.

F. Take a triangular section from the front. Divide this section into two strands.

G. Pick up a 1" section on the left side. Cross this section over the left strand and add it to the right strand.

H. Place both strands in the right hand, index finger in between and palm up.

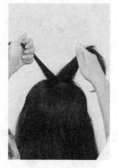 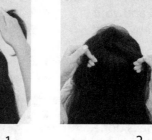 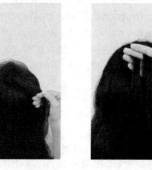

_____ 1.   _____ 2.   _____ 3.

 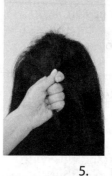 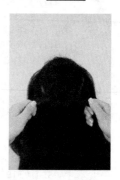

_____ 4.   _____ 5.   _____ 6.

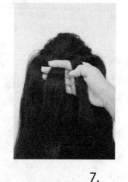 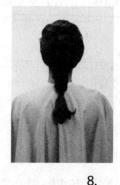

_____ 7.   _____ 8.

38. What do the terms single braids, box braids, and individual braids refer to?

_____

_____

39. The partings or subsections for single braids can be: _____ , _____ ,

or _____ .

40. When determining the direction of the braid, you should braid: _____

_____

41. Extensions for single braids come in a wide range of sizes and lengths and are integrated into the

natural hair using the _____ technique.

42. Fiber for extensions can be derived from: _____ , _____ , or

_____ .

43. Describe how to prepare extension fibers for use.

a) _____

b) _____

c) _____

_____

44. List all the implements and materials needed to complete a single braid without extensions.

a) _____   d) _____

b) _____   e) _____

c) _____   f) _____

45. Match the following descriptions with the photo they describe:

A. Finish each braid by using a rubber band to hold the hair.

B. Divide the hair in half by parting from ear to ear across the crown. Clip away the front section.

C. Part a diagonal section in the back of the head about 1" wide, taking into account the texture and length of the client's hair.

D. Repeat braiding procedure until the back is completed. Repeat in the front section.

E. Divide the section into three even strands. Place your fingers close to the base. Cross the left strand under the center strand and then cross the right strand under. Pass the outer strands under the center strands, moving down the braid to the end.

F. Move to the next section. Repeat the braiding movement by passing the alternating outside strands under the center strand. Keep an even tension on all strands.

_____ 1.   _____ 2.   _____ 3.

_____ 4.   _____ 5.   _____ 6.

46. Match the following descriptions with the photo they describe.

A. As you get closer to the hairline, be aware of the amount of extension hair that is applied to the hairline.

B. Select the appropriate amount of extension fibers from the drawing board. Then fold the fibers in half.

C. Do not add excessive amounts of fiber into a fragile hairline. The fiber should always be proportionate to the hair it is being applied to.

D. The next section should be above the previous section on a diagonal part, moving toward the ear.

E. Part a diagonal section in the back of the head at about a 45-degree angle, from the ear to the nape of the neck.

F. Divide the natural hair into three equal sections. Place the folded extension on top of the natural hair, on the outside and center portions of the braid.

G. Once the back is finished, create a diagonal or horizontal parting above the ear in the front.

H. Finish the ends by spraying water to activate the wave in human hair extensions.

I. Using vertical parts to separate the base into subsections create a diamond-shaped base.

J. Once the extension is in place, begin the underhand braiding movement and braid to the desired length.

K. Part the hair across the crown from ear to ear. Clip away the front section.

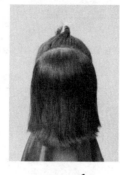
_____ 1.

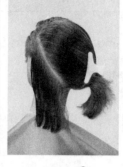
_____ 2.

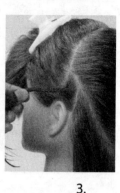
_____ 3.

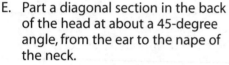
_____ 4.

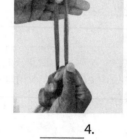
_____ 5.

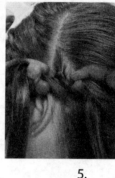
_____ 6.

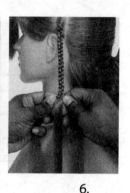
_____ 7.

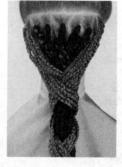
_____ 8.

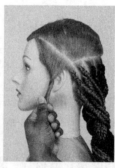
_____ 9.

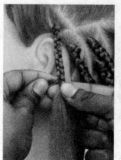
_____ 10.

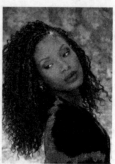
_____ 11.

47. What are cornrows or canerows?

_____

48. Who wears cornrows?

_____

_____

49. How long can cornrows last?

_____

_____

50. What is the feed-in method of applying extensions to cornrows or individual braids?

_____

_____

51. Match the following descriptions with the photo they describe.

A. Pick up a strand from the scalp with each revolution and add it to the outer strand before crossing it under, alternating the side of the braid on which you pick up the hair.

B. Repeat until all the hair is braided. Apply oil sheen for a finished look.

C. Braid to the ends and finish the cornrow; small rubber bands can be used to hold the ends in place.

D. Divide the panel into three even strands. Place your fingers close to the base. Cross the left strand (1) under the center strand (2). Center strand (2) is now on the left and strand (1) is the new center.

E. Determine the correct size and direction of the cornrow base, and use your tail comb to part the hair into two-inch sections and apply a light essential oil to the scalp. Massage the oil throughout the scalp and hair.

F. Create a panel, by taking two even partings to form a neat row for the cornrow base. With a tail comb,

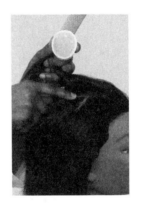

_____ 1.

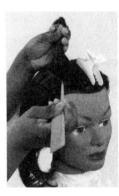

_____ 2.

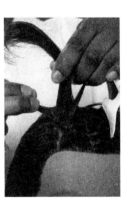

_____ 3.

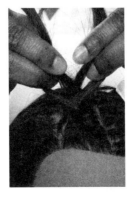

_____ 4.

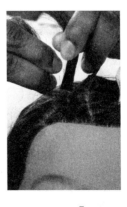

_____ 5.

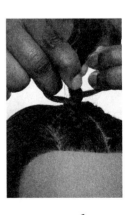

_____ 6.

(continued)

part the hair into a panel, using butterfly clips to keep the other hair pinned to either side.

G. Cross the right strand (3) under the center strand (1). Passing the outer strands under the center strand this way creates the underhand cornrow braid.

H. With each crossing under, or revolution, pick up from the base of the panel a new strand of equal size and add it to the outer strand before crossing it under the center strand.

I. Braid the next panel in the same direction and in the same manner. Keep the partings clean and even.

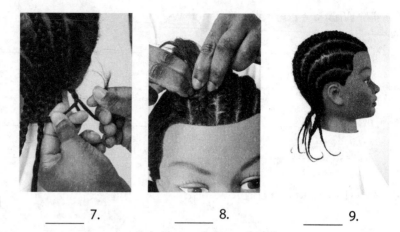

_____ 7.   _____ 8.   _____ 9.

52. Match the following descriptions of braiding cornrows with extensions with the photo they describe.

A. Continue picking up natural hair with each revolution in order to execute the cornrow.

B. Part off a cornrow base in the desired direction.

C. After several revolutions and pick-ups of the natural hair, introduce small amounts of extension fiber, perhaps 10 to 20 fibers. Fold the fibers in the middle and tuck the point in between two adjoining strands of natural hair.

D. On the second revolution, the right strand (3) crosses under strand (1). Pick up a small portion of natural hair and add it to the outer strand during the revolution.

E. With the first revolution, cross strand (1) under strand (2).

F. Repeat until all the hair is braided.

G. The folded fibers will form two portions, which are added to the center and outer strands before the next pick-up and revolution.

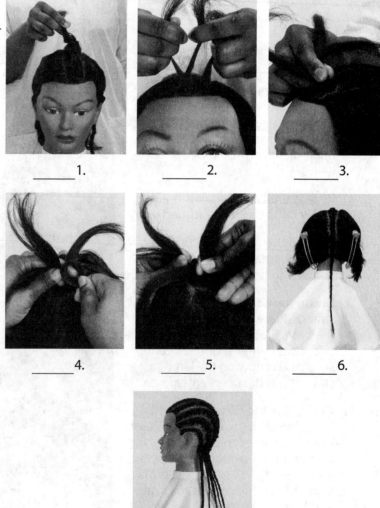

_____ 1.   _____ 2.   _____ 3.

_____ 4.   _____ 5.   _____ 6.

_____ 7.

53. What is hair locking?

_____

_____

54. What are the three basic methods of locking?

a) _____

b) _____

c) _____

55. Describe the comb technique.

_____

_____

_____

56. Describe the palm roll.

_____

_____

_____

57. Describe locking using braids or extensions.

_____

_____

58. Match the following stages of locks with its proper description.

_____ 1. Phase 1, Pre-lock Stage   A. Lock is totally closed at the end. Hair is tightly meshed

_____ 2. Phase 2, Sprouting Stage   B. Hair is soft and is coiled into spiral configurations.

_____ 3. Phase 3, Growing Stage   C. After several years of maturation, the lock may start to weaken
                                            or come apart at the ends

_____ 4. Phase 4, Maturation Stage   D. A bulb can be felt at the end of each lock. Hair begins to
                                            regain length. Locks are closed at the ends, dense and dull,
                                            not reflecting any light.

_____ 5. Phase 5, Atrophy Stage   E. Hair begins to interlace and mesh.

14

WIGS AND HAIR ENHANCEMENTS

Date: _____

Rating:_____

Test Pages: 457-483

POINT TO PONDER:

"Common sense is the knack of seeing things as they are, and doing things as they ought to be done."—Stowe

1. What role did wigs play in ancient Egypt?

   _____

   _____

2. Why did men wear wigs in 18th-century England?

   _____

3. Who wears wigs today?

   _____

THE CONSULTATION

4. What things should be discussed during the client consultation for wig services?

   a) _____

   b) _____

   c) _____

5. List some of the most common reasons a client may want to try a hair enhancement.

   a) _____

   b) _____

   c) _____

WIGS

6. A _____ can be defined as an artificial covering for the head consisting of a

   network of interwoven hair.

7. When wearing a wig, the client's hair is concealed _____ .

   a) partially

   b) in the nape

   c) completely

   d) in the crown

8. If a hair addition does not fully cover the head, it is classified as a _____ , which is a

   small wig used to cover the top or crown of the head.

9. What is the fastest way to tell if a strand of hair is a synthetic product or real human hair?

   _____

   _____

   _____

10. List the advantages of human hair wigs.

    a) _____

    b) _____

    c) _____

    d) _____

    e) _____

    f) _____

11. Can a human hair wig react to the climate the way natural hair does?

    _____

    _____

12. A human hair wig never needs to be reset because it always retains its original style.

_____ True

_____ False

13. The color of a human hair wig will oxidize, meaning that it will fade with exposure to light.

_____ True

_____ False

14. Human hair wigs are so strong that the hair will not break or split if mistreated by harsh brushing, back-combing, or excessive use of heat.

_____ True

_____ False

15. Which synthetic fibers have been so greatly improved that they can often fool stylists into thinking they are natural fibers?

a) _____   b) _____

16. What is one of the greatest advantages of synthetic wigs?

_____

17. Which is more expensive to purchase, a human hair wig or a synthetic wig?

_____

18. You will need to reset a synthetic wig every time you shampoo it.

_____ True

_____ False

19. How are most synthetic ready-to-wear wigs styled?

_____

20. There is no additional work ever needed on a synthetic, ready-to-wear wig.

_____ True

_____ False

21. What colors are synthetic wigs available in?

_____

_____

22. Is there any difference in the color quality of the wigs?

_____

_____

23. Synthetic colors will fade and oxidize when exposed to long periods in the sun.

_____ True

_____ False

24. Synthetic hair cannot be exposed to extreme heat such as curling irons, hot rollers, or the high heat of blow-dryers.

_____ True

_____ False

25. Is it advisable to color synthetic fibers?

_____

26. What is a telltale sign that a wig is made of synthetic fiber?

_____

27. What is the one thing to remember about a wig's quality?

_____

_____

28. Wigs made of European hair are the most inexpensive wigs.

_____ True

_____ False

29. Of all human hair wigs which are more expensive—virgin hair or color-treated hair?

_____

30. What regions of the world are the largest providers of human hair for commercial purposes?

_____ a) India and South America

_____ b) Middle East

_____ c) Asia and North America

_____ d) India and Asia

31. Indian hair is usually available in lengths from _____ inches.

a) 3 to 7

b) 8 to 12

c) 12 to 16

d) 17 to 22

32. Asian hair is available in lengths of _____ inches.

a) 12 to 18

b) 12 to 24

c) 12 to 26

d) 12 to 28

33. Indian hair is naturally _____ while Asian hair is naturally _____ .

34. Is human hair ever mixed with any other fiber in a wig? What kind of fibers?

_____

35. What type of animal fibers would be mixed with human hair in wigs?

_____

36. Where are mixed-hair products most often used?

_____ a) In hair competitions

_____ b) For cancer patients

_____ c) In theatrical settings

_____ d) For bridal updos

37. When selecting a wig for the client you must first ask:

    _____

38. Next you will need to know if the hair has been _____ or is _____.

39. If the hair is human hair, you will need to determine if it is graded in terms of _____,

    _____, and _____.

40. What is turned hair?

    _____

    _____

41. What is fallen hair?

    _____

    _____

42. If the cuticle has been removed from the hair, this often means you cannot _____

    the hair, because it will tend to _____.

43. What is a reasonable amount of time for a wig to hold up if a client is maintaining her wig at home, herself?

    _____

44. Name the two basic categories of wigs.

    a) _____

    b) _____

45. How are cap wigs constructed?

    _____

46. Are cap wigs made with a one-size-fits-all mentality?

    _____

47. What does it mean if a cap wig is hand-knotted?

    _____

48. How are cap wigs fitted to the head?

_____

_____

_____

49. How are capless wigs made?

_____

50. What is a weft?

_____

51. Like the cap wig, a capless wig entirely covers the head.

_____ True

_____ False

52. What type of wig is pictured in the illustration below?

_____

53. What type of client should use a cap wig?

_____

54. Which type of wig is healthier?

_____

55. What are hand-tied or hand-knotted wigs?

_____

_____

56. Where in the wig is hand tying most often done?

_____

57. What is the advantage of hand knotting?

_____

58. The hand-tied method most closely resembles actual human hair growth, with flexibility at the roots.

_____ True

_____ False

59. What are semi-hand-tied wigs?

_____

60. What are the advantages of semi-hand-tied wigs?

a) _____   c) _____

b) _____

61. What are machine-made wigs and how are they constructed?

_____

_____

62. Are there any disadvantages to machine-made wigs?

_____

63. Are there any advantages to machine-made wigs?

_____

64. Why is it important to note the artificial growth patterns of a wig?

_____

65. The most flexible and versatile growth patterns is the _____ wig.

66. The least flexible and versatile growth patterns is the _____ wig.

67. Why are machine made wigs so inflexible?

   _____

68. The first thing you need to know when ordering a custom-made wig is

   _____.

69. What implements and materials will you need in order to measure a client for a custom-ordered wig?

   a) _____   d) _____

   b) _____   e) _____

   c) _____

70. What steps should you take to prepare your client for the wig measuring service?

   a) _____

   b) _____

   c) _____

71. What area of the head should you measure first? _____

72. Describe how to accurately measure the circumference of the head.

   _____

   _____

73. Describe the action taking place in this illustration.

   _____

   _____

   _____

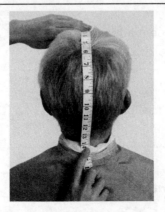

74. What is the next section that should be measured?

_____

75. Measure from ear to ear a second time, this time from _____.

76. Place the tape across the crown and measure from _____.

77. What area of the head is being measured in this illustration?

_____

78. Describe the procedure for cleanup after the measurements are taken.

a) _____

b) _____

c) _____

d) _____

79. Once you have the client's head measurements what should you do with them?

_____

_____

80. List any other information you should send to the wig maker along with the client's head measurements.

_____

81. Are measurements required for a ready-to-wear wig?

_____

82. What is a block?

_____

_____

83. Canvas blocks are available in _____ sizes, from 20" to 22-¹/₂".

   a) Three

   b) Four

   c) Five

   d) Six

84. The block is attached to your work area with a _____, which allows for greater control.

85. When mounting the wig on the block, pin it evenly with T-shaped pins at which points?

   a) _____   c) _____

   b) _____

86. What implements and materials will be needed to prepare the client to put on a wig?

   a) _____   d) _____

   b) _____   e) _____

   c) _____   f) _____

87. How will you drape the client to prepare her to receive the wig?

_____

88. What are the two most common options for preparing the hair prior to putting on the wig?

   a) _____   b) _____

89. What is the procedure for preparing the hair with pin curls.

   a) _____

   b) _____

_____

90. What is the procedure for preparing the hair with a hair wrap?

   a) _____

   b) _____

   c) _____

91. How should you first approach putting the wig on the client?

   _____

   _____

92. How do you fit the wig around the ears?

   _____

93. If the wig is loose, how can you tighten it?

   _____

94. Should you tighten the wig while it's on the clients head?

   _____

95. Describe the extra step you should take if the client has long or thick hair.

   _____

   _____

96. Is extra pinning necessary for clients with thin or short hair?

   _____

97. What is the best way to clean a wig?

   _____

98. If shampooing is recommended, what type of shampoo should you use?

   _____ a) oily hair shampoo

   _____ b) clarifying shampoo

   _____ c) shampoo for color-treated hair

   _____ d) shampoo for dandruff

99. When cutting a wig, your goal is to make the hair look more _____.

100. How can a stylist achieve a natural look when cutting a wig?

_____

_____

101. When cutting and trimming wigs what basic methods of haircutting should you follow?

_____

_____

102. What is free-form cutting on a wig?

_____

103. After free-form cutting you should style the wig on:

_____ a) the block

_____ b) the client's head

_____ c) yourself

_____ d) another client

104. Free-form cutting is usually done on wet hair, which allows you to see more easily how the hair will fall.

_____ True

_____ False

105. When using heat on a human hair wig, always set the styling tool to what position?

_____ a) off

_____ b) low

_____ c) medium

_____ d) high

106. The best type of brush to use on a wig made of natural hair is one with _____.

107. What type of styling products should be used on a human hair wig?

_____

108. Where should coloring, perming, setting, and basic cut outlining be done on a wig?

_____

109. The combing-out and finishing touches for most contemporary cuts should be completed on the

_____ in order to achieve proper balance and personalization.

110. In order for a wig to look natural and believable these areas must appear the most convincing:

a) _____

b) _____

c) _____

111. To style the wig to look as natural as possible always follow the

_____ .

112. To make the hairline look natural, you should _____ gently, as the fluffy effect softens

the hairline.

113. You should release the client's hair around the hairline and cut and blend it into the wig hair.

_____ True

_____ False

114. What is the "wind test" and how is it achieved?

_____

_____

_____

115. When styling a wig, you should make the final result look perfect.

_____ True

_____ False

116. How will you know for sure if the wig you've just styled has the right look for the client?

_____

117. What colors are most commercially available wigs?

_____

118. If you are going to custom-color the hair, you should use hair that has been _____

_____ .

119. If you are planning on coloring a wig, you must first check to see if the _____ is intact.

120. Hair in which the cuticle is absent is very _____ and will react to color in an extreme manner.

121. Always _____ the hair prior to full color application.

    a) patch test

    b) decolorize

    c) strand test

    d) perm

122. When coloring a wig which color products are best to use?

    a) _____   d) _____

    b) _____   e) _____

    c) _____

123. What type of color can be used on human hair wigs with good porosity?

_____

124. If a human hair wig is porous, what type of color should you use?

_____

125. When coloring a human hair wig or hairpiece, conduct regular color checks every_____minutes.

    a) 1 to 2

    b) 5 to 10

    c) 15 to 20

    d) 25 to 30

126. If you want to perm a human hair wig hair to match the client's natural wave pattern, you need to know how the hair was _____.

127. You may safely perm wig hair that has been colored with a metallic dye.

_____ True

_____ False

128. Where should the wig be while performing the perm?

_____

HAIRPIECES

129. What is a hairpiece and how much coverage does it give?

_____

_____

130. How are hairpieces used?

_____

131. Where must a headpiece be placed on the head?

_____

132. Name the temporary attachment methods used to affix hairpieces.

a) _____   d) _____

b) _____   e) _____

c) _____

133. An_____ has an opening in the base through which the client's own hair is pulled to blend with the hair of the hairpiece.

134. Integration hairpieces are a very lightweight and natural-looking and are used to _____ and_____ to the client's hair.

135. What type of client is ideally suited for an integration hairpiece?

_____

136. A _____ is a small wig used to cover the top and crown of the head.

137. Only men use toupees.

_____ True

_____ False

138. How are toupees attached?

_____

_____

139. _____ hairpieces are a great salon product for special occasions or for use as fashion accessories.

140. Fashion hairpieces vary in _____ and are constructed on a _____.

141. Fashion hairpieces are attached on a temporary basis using:

_____.

142. In order to achieve a natural look, it is crucial that you _____ the client's hair with the hairpiece.

HAIR EXTENSIONS

143. What are hair extensions and why are they used?

_____

_____

144. Hair extensions are removed each evening before bedtime.

_____ True

_____ False

145. How far away from the front hairline, sides, and nape should hair extensions be attached?

_____ a) ½"

_____ b) 1"

_____ c) 2"

_____ d) 5"

146. When working with curly hair you must decide if you are _____ or adding another curl pattern to the hair.

147. In the _____ method, hair extensions are secured at the base of the client's own hair by sewing.

148. In the track and sew method the hair is attached to an _____, which serves as the track.

149. The _____ of the track determines how the hair will fall.

    a) pitch

    b) angle

    c) cut

    d) length

150. In what direction are tracks positioned?

    _____

    _____

    _____

    _____

151. How are the sizes of the sections determined?

    _____

152. How are the extensions sewn onto a track?

    _____

153. Name the stitches that may be used to sew the extension to the track.

    a) _____   c) _____

    b) _____

154. _____ involves attaching hair wefts or single strands with an adhesive or a glue gun.

155. How long will the bonded hair last?

_____ a) one to two weeks

_____ b) two to four weeks

_____ c) four to six weeks

_____ d) six to eight weeks

156. What factors affect how long the hair will remain bonded?

a) _____   c) _____

b) _____

157. Describe the procedure for bonding extensions.

a) _____

b) _____

c) _____

d) _____

e) _____

f) _____

g) _____

158. How are bonded wefts removed?

_____

159. What is the method in which the extension is bonded to the client's own hair with a bonding material that is activated by heat from a special tool?

_____

160. What are the advantages of the fusion method?

a) _____

_____

b) _____

_____

c) _____

_____

161. How long do fused extensions last?

_____

162. Why is fusion a good choice for clients with fine, limp hair?

_____

163. The fusion procedure involves wrapping a _____ strip around both the client's hair

and the extension.

164. Describe the action that allows the extension to be fused:

_____

_____

15
CHEMICAL TEXTURE SERVICES

Date: _____

Rating:_____

Text Pages: 485-543

POINT TO PONDER:

"Minds are like parachutes—they only function when open."—Thomas Dewar

1. What do chemical texture services cause?

   _____

2. Texture services can be used to _____ straight hair, _____ overly curly hair, or

   _____ coarse, straight hair and make it more pliable and easier to work with.

3. Texture services include:

   a) _____   c) _____

   b) _____

PERMANENT WAVING

4. Permanent waving is a two-step process involving:

   _____.

5. What is responsible for the physical change?

   _____

6. What is responsible for the chemical change?

   _____

7. In permanent waving, the size, shape, and type of curl are determined by the

   _____.

8. Does the strength of the permanent waving solution cause the hair to curl any more than water causes a wet set to curl?

_____

_____

9. What function does wetting the hair before wrapping it in perm rods serve?

_____

_____

10. What is the major difference between a wet set and a permanent wave?

_____

11. What type of bonds are broken in the perm process?

_____

12. Wrapping the hair on small tools or rods increases the tension, which

_____ a) decreases the amount of curl

_____ b) relaxes the curl

_____

_____ d) elongates the curl

13. What can happen if a curl is wound with too much tension?

_____

14. All perm wraps begin by sectioning the hair into _____.

15. How do you determine the size, shape, and direction of these panels?

_____

16. Each panel is further divided into subsections called _____.

17. The size of each base section is usually the _____ and _____ of the tool being used.

18. _____ refers to the position of the tool in relation to its base section and is

determined by the angle at which the hair is wrapped.

19. Tools can be wrapped

   a) _____   c) _____

   b) _____

20. Identify the type of placement illustrated below _____ .

21. The on-base placement requires that the hair be wrapped at an angle of _____ degrees beyond

   perpendicular to its base section.

   a) 15

   b) 30

   c) 45

   d) 60

22. On-base placement will result in greater volume at the _____ area.

   a) mid-shaft

   b) hair ends

   c) scalp

   d) cuticle

23. _____ placement refers to wrapping the hair at an angle of 90 degrees to its

   base section.

24. Where is the tool positioned in a half-off-base placement?

   _____

25. The half-off-base placement maximizes stress and tension on the hair.

   _____ True

   _____ False

26. _____ refers to wrapping the hair at an angle 45 degrees below

perpendicular to its base section.

27. Off-base placement creates the most amount of volume and results in a curl pattern that begins farthest away from the scalp.

_____ True

_____ False

28. The angle at which the tool is positioned on the head—horizontally, vertically, or diagonally—is called

_____.

29. _Base direction_ also refers to the directional pattern in which the hair is _____.

30. What direction of wrapping causes the least amount of stress to the hair?

_____

31. Wrapping against the natural growth pattern causes excess stress that may _____

the hair.

    a) curl or condition

    b) cut or elongate

    c) damage or break

    d) curl or dry

32. Name the two basic methods of wrapping the hair around the perm tool.

    a) _____   b) _____

33. In _____ the hair strands are wrapped from the ends to the scalp, in

overlapping layers.

34. In croquignole perms the hair is wrapped at an angle _____ to the length

of the tool.

35. Where is each new layer of hair placed?

_____

36. Croquignole wraps increase the effective size of the tool with each new overlapping layer and produce a

    _____ at the ends and a _____ curl at the scalp.

37. How are spiral perms wound?

    _____

38. Is there any difference in the finished curl?

    _____

39. At what angle are spiral perms wrapped?

    _____

40. The angle at which the hair is wrapped causes the hair to _____

    like the grip on a tennis racquet.

41. The spiral wrap has what effect on the size of the curl?

    _____

42. Name the four types of rods that are commonly used for perming.

    a) _____   c) _____

    b) _____   d) _____

43. Which is the most common type of perm rod?

    _____

44. Which wrapping technique are concave rods usually used with?

    _____

45. Describe the structure of a concave rod.

    _____

46. What kind of curl do concave rods produce?

    _____

47. _____ are usually used with a croquignole wrapping technique.

48. How do straight rods differ from croquignole rods?

_____

_____

49. Concave and straight rods come in different lengths.

_____ True

_____ False

50. What factor determines if a long straight rod can also be used with a spiral wrapping technique to produce spiral perms?

_____

51. Why are short rods used and where?

_____

_____

52. _____ are usually about 12 inches long with a uniform diameter

along the entire length.

53. What is a soft bender rod made of and why is it useful?

_____

54. What wrapping techniques are soft bender rods used for?

_____

55. The_____ is ideal for spiral wrapping on _____ .

56. How is the circle tool secured after the hair is wrapped?

_____

57. What are end papers or end wraps and how are they used?

_____

_____

58. Where are end papers placed?

_____

_____

59. Name the most common end paper techniques.

   a) _____   c) _____

   b) _____

60. Identify each of the end wrap techniques illustrated below.

_____   _____   _____

61. The_____ uses two end papers, one placed under and one over the strand

   of hair being wrapped.

62. The double flat wrap provides the_____ control over the hair ends and helps keep them

   evenly distributed over the entire length of the tool.

63. The_____ is similar to the double flat wrap, but uses only one end paper,

   placed over the top of the strand of hair being wrapped.

64. The_____ uses one end paper folded in half over the hair ends like an

   envelope.

65. When using the bookend wrap be careful to _____

   and_____.

SAFETY PRECAUTIONS

66. It is okay to give a permanent to any client who has experienced an allergic reaction to a previous permanent.

   _____ True

   _____ False

67. You may save opened or unused waving lotion or neutralizer for use on your next client.

   _____ True

   _____ False

68. Do not dilute or add anything to the waving lotion or neutralizer unless specified in the manufacturer's directions.

   _____ True

   _____ False

69. If waving lotion accidentally gets into the client's eyes or on the client's skin, rinse thoroughly with warm water.

   _____ True

   _____ False

70. As long as you are familiar with a perm product, you may feel free to experiment with it.

   _____ True

   _____ False

71. Wear gloves when applying solutions if you know you have airborne allergies.

   _____ True

   _____ False

72. Immediately replace cotton or towels that have become wet with waving solution.

   _____ True

   _____ False

73. If you are familiar with your client's hair and scalp, there is no need to examine the scalp each time you perform a perm service.

_____ True

_____ False

74. If using a conditioning perm solution it is okay to perm hair that is excessively damaged or shows signs of breakage.

_____ True

_____ False

75. Do not attempt to perm hair that has been previously treated with hydroxide relaxers.

_____ True

_____ False

76. Always perform a test for metallic salts if there is a possibility that metallic haircolor was used on the hair previously.

_____ True

_____ False

77. If a client has allergies, you should always apply protective barrier cream around the client's hairline and ears prior to applying permanent waving solution.

_____ True

_____ False

78. How can the presence of metallic salts in the hair affect a perm?

_____

_____

79. Where are metallic salts commonly found?

_____

80. What types of haircolors for home use usually contain metallic salts?

_____

_____

81. List the steps involved in testing for metallic salts

a) _____

b) _____

c) _____

_____

PERMANENT WAVING PROCEDURES

82. The basic perm wrap is also called a _____ .

83. In the basic perm wrap _____ the tools within a panel move in the same direction and are

positioned on equal size bases.

a) none

b) some

c) a few

d) all

84. In the basic perm wrap all base sections are _____ , with the same length and width

as the perm tool, and the base control is _____ base.

85. In the _____ , the movement curves within sectioned-out panels.

86. What shape sections are used in the wrapping of the curvature perm wrap?

_____

87. The_____ has base sections that are offset from each other row by row, to

prevent noticeable splits and to blend the flow of the hair.

88. Name the various starting points of different bricklay patterns.

_____

89. Why are the starting points important?

_____

90. The_____ uses zigzag partings to divide base areas.

91. When would you use the weave technique?

_____

_____

92. The double tool perm technique is also called a _____ because two tools are

used for one strand of hair, one on top of the other.

93. How is the piggyback wrap done?

_____

_____

94. What effect does the piggyback wrap usually produce?

_____

_____

95. The _____ wrap is done at an angle that causes the hair to spiral along

the length of the tool.

96. What occurs if the layers in a spiral perm partially overlap as they go along?

_____

_____

97. What kind of curl is produced by the spiral wrap?

_____

98. What types of rods can be used for a spiral wrap?

_____

99. Why do you need to take preliminary test curls?

_____

100. Preliminary test curls provide the following information.

   a) _____

   b) _____

   c) _____

101. List all of the implements and materials you need to perform a perm service.

a) _____   k) _____

b) _____   l) _____

c) _____   m) _____

d) _____   n) _____

e) _____   o) _____

f) _____   p) _____

g) _____   q) _____

h) _____   r) _____

i) _____   s) _____

j) _____   t) _____

102. How do you prepare yourself for the perm service?

_____

103. How do you prepare your client for the perm service?

a) _____

b) _____

c) _____

d) _____

e) _____

f) _____

104. When doing a preliminary test curl how many curls should you wrap and where should they be?

_____

105. It isn't necessary to wrap a coil of cotton around each tool when performing the preliminary test.

_____ True

_____ False

106. After waving lotion is applied to the wrapped curls how long should you wait before checking on the curl?

_____

107. How do you check each test curl for proper curl development?

_____

108. How do you know if the curl development is complete?

_____

109. Once the curl has been formed, apply the neutralizer.

_____ True

_____ False

110. For how long should you rinse perm solution from the hair?

_____ a) one minute
_____ b) three minutes
_____ c) five minutes
_____ d) seven minutes

111. After rinsing you must _____ the hair thoroughly before applying the neutralizer.

112. How long should you allow the neutralizer to process?

_____

113. If the test curls are extremely damaged or overprocessed you should:

_____ a) re-perm them
_____ b) proceed with the perm service
_____ c) condition them before proceeding with the perm service
_____ d) do not proceed with the perm service

Procedure for Basic Perm Wrap

114. How many panels should the hair be divided into for the basic perm wrap?

_____

115. How wide should the panels be?

_____

116. Hair should be wet when you begin to wrap and dry when you finish.

_____ True

_____ False

117. Begin wrapping at the _____ by making _____ partings the same size as the tool.

118. What angle should the hair be held at to wrap?

_____ a) 15 degrees
_____ b) 30 degrees
_____ c) 45 degrees
_____ d) 90 degrees

119. Using _____ end papers roll the hair down to the scalp and position the tool half off base.

a) one
b) two
c) three
d) four

120. How should the band be fastened across the top of the tool?

_____

121. How are roller picks used?

_____

122. Before you begin processing the perm you must apply protective barrier cream to the _____ and around the _____ .

123. After the cream, apply _____ around the entire hairline and offer the client a towel to blot any drips.

124. What position should the client be in when you apply the waving lotion to the back area?

_____

125. What position should the client be in when you apply the waving lotion to the front and side areas?

_____

126. What do you use to apply the waving lotion?

_____

127. How well saturated should each tool be?

_____

128. If a plastic cap is used, how should you prepare it for the client?

_____

129. If during processing cotton and towels become saturated with solution you should:

_____ a) leave them undisturbed until the perm is processed
_____ b) spray them with water to stop the lotion from processing
_____ c) spray them with neutralizer to stop the lotion from processing
_____ d) replace them with clean dry cotton and towels

130. Although you should always process the perm according to the manufacturer's directions, a good rule of thumb for processing is that it usually takes _____ at room temperature.

a) less than 10 minutes

b) less than 20 minutes

c) more than 20 minutes

d) less than 30 minutes

130. How do you know when the perm has processed?

_____

131. When processing is completed, rinse the hair thoroughly for at least _____ minutes, then towel-blot the hair on each tool to remove any excess moisture.

132. If the product you are using recommends that you apply a pre-neutralizing conditioner to the hair, when is this done?

_____

133. How is neutralizer applied?

_____

134. How long should you allow the neutralizer to stay on the hair?

_____

135. After the neutralizer has processed, you should apply any unused product to the hair and wait five more minutes before removing the rods.

_____ True

_____ False

136. After the tools are removed from the hair, you should_____

and style as desired.

137. How do you clean up after the perm service?

a) _____

b) _____

c) _____

d) _____

e) _____

Procedure for Curvature Perm Wrap

138. Where do you begin sectioning for the curvature perm wrap?

_____

139. How large should the sections be?

_____

_____

140. Should you section the panels in advance?

_____

_____

141. Describe wrapping the section.

a) _____

b) _____

c) _____

d) _____

142. The remaining base sections in the panel should be _____ on the outside of the panel, the side farthest away from the face.

    a) thinner

    b) wider

    c) longer

    d) shorter

143. When you reach the last rod at the hairline, what should you do?

_____

144. After you have wrapped panel one, continue to panel two. Where is panel two?

_____

145. Where is the third panel?

_____

146. Where is the fourth panel?

_____

147. All panels should fit the_____ of the head and should _____ the surrounding panels.

Procedure for Bricklay Perm Wrap

148. How is the hair sectioned for the bricklay wrap?

_____

_____

149. What is the base direction?

_____

150. Hold the hair at a _____ degree angle to the head and using two end papers, roll the hair down to the scalp and position the rod half-off-base.

151. In the second row, which is directly _____ , part out two base sections for two rods offset from the center of the first rod.

152. Hold the hair at a 90-degree angle to the head and, using _____ end papers, roll the hair down to the scalp and position the rods half-off-base.

153. How should you begin the third row?

    _____

154. Continue to part out rows that _____ around the curve of the head through the crown area.

155. When do you stop curving the rows?

    _____

156. To complete the wrap you use _____ throughout the back of the head.

Procedure for Weave Technique

157. The weave technique can be used only with the bricklay wrapping technique.

    _____ True

    _____ False

158. What size should the base section be?

    _____

159. How is the zigzag parting made?

    _____

160. Using two end papers, roll the _____ half of the strand down to the scalp, and comb the _____ half of the base section and roll the strand down to the scalp

Procedure for Double Tool (Piggyback) Technique

161. With which wrapping patterns can the double tool (piggyback) technique be used?

    _____

162. Describe how to wrap the piggyback wrap.

a) _____

_____

b) _____

_____

c) _____

_____

d) _____

_____

e) _____

_____

163. Depending on the length and size of the rods, it may be possible to roll as many as _____

end strands together on the same end rod.

a) three

b) four

c) five

d) six

Procedure for Spiral Perm Wrap

164. Where on the head do you begin with the spiral wrap?

_____

165. How many panels is the hair parted into?

_____

166. How are the first four panels parted?

_____

167. Where is the fifth panel located?

_____

168. Where do you begin to wrap?

_____

169. Describe how to wrap the first spiral curl.

a) _____

_____

b) _____

_____

c) _____

_____

d) _____

_____

e) _____

_____

f) _____

_____

170. When you begin to wrap the second row above and parallel to the first row, you will begin wrapping at

the _____ side from the side where the first row began, and move in the direction

_____ the direction established in the first row.

171. Follow the same procedure to wrap the remaining rows beginning to wrap each tool at the same end established in the previous row.

_____ True

_____ False

Partial Perms

172. What is a partial perm?

_____

173. Partial perms can be used for:

a) _____

b) _____

c) _____

174. How can you make a smooth transition from the rolled section to the unrolled section?

_____

175. What can happen if waving lotion is applied to unrolled hair during a partial perm?

_____

176. How can you protect the unrolled hair?

_____

Perms for Men

177. For what reasons do male clients request perms?

_____

178. What problems can a perm help a male client with?

_____

_____

179. Are the techniques for permanent waving men's hair different than those used for women?

_____

CHEMICAL HAIR RELAXERS

180. Chemical hair relaxing is the process of _____ the basic structure of extremely

curly hair into a straight form.

181. Whereas permanent waving _____ straight hair, chemical hair relaxing _____

curly hair.

182. In what ways are chemical relaxing and permanent waving similar?

_____

183. In what ways are chemical relaxing and permanent waving dissimilar?

_____

184. All chemical relaxers change the shape of the hair by breaking disulfide bonds.

_____ True

_____ False

CHEMICAL HAIR RELAXING PROCEDURES

185. The steps for hydroxide relaxers are different from those for thio relaxers.

_____ True

_____ False

186. Although all hydroxide relaxers follow the same procedure, different application methods are used for

_____ relaxers and _____ relaxers.

187. A _____ relaxer application should be used for hair that has not had previous

chemical texture services.

188. Why does a virgin relaxer start $\frac{1}{4}$ to $\frac{1}{2}$ inch away from the scalp?

_____

_____

189. To avoid overprocessing and scalp irritation, do not apply relaxer to the hair closest to the _____

or to the _____ until the last few minutes of processing.

190. A _____ relaxer application should be used for hair that has had previous chemical

texture services.

191. The application for a retouch relaxer starts $\frac{1}{4}$ to $\frac{1}{2}$ inch away from the scalp and includes

_____ .

    a) only the previously relaxed hair.

    b) only the previously permed hair.

    c) only the new growth

    d) only the old hair.

192. To avoid overprocessing and scalp irritation, _____
_____ .

193. If the previously relaxed hair requires additional straightening you should apply

_____ a) pressing oil and a cream base
_____ b) relaxer for the last few minutes of processing
_____ c) neutralizer to the regrowth
_____ d) perming lotion to the hair ends

194. What is a normalizing solution?

_____

_____

195. How do you know if the hair is sufficiently relaxed?

_____

196. How is a strand test done?

_____

_____

_____

197. What factors influence the processing time?

a) _____

b) _____

c) _____

198. List the implements and materials you need for relaxing with hydroxide relaxer.

a) _____   h) _____

b) _____   i) _____

c) _____   j) _____

d) _____   k) _____

e) _____   l) _____

f) _____   m) _____

g) _____   n) _____

199. How do you prepare yourself and your client for the relaxing procedure?

a) _____

b) _____

c) _____

d) _____

e) _____

f) _____

200. Should you shampoo the client's hair prior to a hydroxide relaxer? Why or why not?

_____

201. Into how many sections should the hair be parted when applying virgin hydroxide relaxers?

_____

202. Where is protective base cream applied?

_____

203. Should protective base cream be applied to the entire scalp?

_____

204. It isn't necessary to wear gloves during the relaxer procedure.

_____ True

_____ False

205. Begin application in the most resistant area, usually at the _____.

206. Make_____ inch horizontal partings and apply the relaxer to the top of the strand first, then to

the underside

a) $\frac{1}{8}$ to $\frac{1}{4}$

b) $\frac{1}{4}$ to $\frac{1}{2}$

c) ($\frac{1}{2}$ to $\frac{3}{4}$)

d) ($\frac{3}{4}$ to one)

207. What may be used to apply the relaxer?

_____

208. Apply relaxer ¼ to ½ inch away from the scalp and up to the _____ .

   a) midshaft

   b) porous ends

   c) the previously relaxed hair

   d) halfway point

209. To avoid scalp irritation

_____ .

210. After the relaxer has been applied to all sections, use the back of the comb or your hands to

_____ .

211. Processing usually takes _____ at room temperature.

   a) less than 10 minutes

   b) less than 20 minutes

   c) more than 20 minutes

   d) less than 30 minutes

212. During the last few minutes of processing.

   _____ a) remove all of the relaxer as quickly as possible
   _____ b) work the relaxer down to the scalp and through the ends of the hair
   _____ c) rinse the hair immediately
   _____ d) spray the hair with water to stop the action of the relaxer

213. How should you remove all of the relaxer?

_____

214. In the neutralization procedure for hydroxide relaxers how many times should you shampoo with an acid-balanced neutralizing shampoo?

    _____ a) no shampooing is needed
    _____ b) at least one time
    _____ c) at least two times
    _____ d) at least three times

215. If you are using a neutralizing shampoo with a color indicator, a change in color indicates

    _____

    _____.

216. Another option for removing relaxer is to use a _____.

217. How is a normalizing solution applied?

    _____

    _____

218. After the normalizing solution is applied, what should be done?

    _____

219. Describe the cleanup procedure for all relaxers.

    a) _____

    b) _____

    c) _____

    d) _____

    e) _____

220. When preparing to do a retouch with hydroxide relaxer you should shampoo the hair.

    _____ True

    _____ False

221. Describe how to section the hair.

    _____

    _____

222. Is it necessary to apply a protective base cream? Where?

_____

223. Where should you begin application of the relaxer?

_____

224. For a retouch application where should the relaxer be applied?

_____

225. If you allow the relaxer to overlap what may happen?

_____

226. Describe what the stylist is doing in the illustration below.

_____

227. How long should you allow for the process?

_____

228. During the last few minutes of processing, work the relaxer _____.

229. If the ends of the hair need additional relaxing, when should you work the relaxer through to the ends?

_____

230. The entire process for thio relaxers is the same as for hydroxide relaxers.

_____ True

_____ False.

231. In addition to the implements and materials you would use for hydroxide relaxers, what do you need for a thio process?

   a) _____

   b) _____

   c) _____

232. How should you prepare yourself and your client for a thio relaxer?

   _____

233. To complete the procedure for a virgin thio relaxer you should follow the exact same application procedure as for virgin hydroxide relaxers.

   _____ True

   _____ False

234. After your client's hair has processed, how do you neutralize for thio relaxers?

   a) _____

   _____

   b) _____

   _____

   c) _____

   _____

   d) _____

   _____

SOFT CURL PERMANENTS (CURL RE-FORMING)

235. What is a soft curl permanent?

   _____

236. By what other names is a soft curl permanent called?

   _____

237. What effect does a soft curl permanent have on the hair?

   _____

238. Soft curl permanents use _____ and _____,

just as thio permanent waves do.

239. A soft curl permanent is actually _____ services.

    a) two

    b) three

    c) four

    d) five

240. The first step in a soft curl permanent is to relax extremely curly hair with a _____.

The second step is to_____.

241. When wrapping the hair on tools, all base sections should be _____, with the same

length and width as the perm tool.

242. The base direction should be _____ hair growth.

    a) above the

    b) in the opposite direction to

    c) in the same direction as

    d) below the

243. The base control should be _____ base.

    a) on

    b) off

    c) half-on

    d) half-off

244. Once it is wrapped on large tools, the hair is then processed with a _____

or curl booster.

245. After processing, how is the hair treated?

_____

246. List all the implements and supplies you need for a soft curl perm.

a) _____   l) _____

b) _____   m) _____

c) _____   n) _____

d) _____   o) _____

e) _____   p) _____

f) _____   q) _____

g) _____   r) _____

h) _____   s) _____

i) _____   t) _____

j) _____   u) _____

k) _____   v) _____

247. How do you prepare yourself and your client for a soft curl permanent?

a) _____

b) _____

c) _____

d) _____

248. Should you shampoo your client's hair before beginning the soft curl permanent?

_____

_____

249. The first step in the procedure for a soft curl permanent is to follow the procedure for applying

_____.

250. After the hair has processed and is rinsed, part the hair into _____ panels.

a) six

b) eight

c) nine

d) ten

251. Use the length of the _____ to measure the width of the panels.

252. Where should you begin wrapping the head?

_____

253. Apply and distribute the thio curl booster to each _____ as you wrap the hair.

254. What size should the horizontal parting be?

_____

255. Hold the hair at a _____ angle to the head.

    a) 15-degree

    b) 30-degree

    c) 45-degree

    d) 90-degree

256. Using _____ end papers, roll the hair down to the scalp and position the rod half-off-base.

    a) two

    b) three

    c) four

    d) five

257. Can roller picks be used?

_____

258. After the entire head is wrapped, place cotton around the _____ and _____

and apply _____ to all the curls until they are completely saturated.

259. If a plastic cap is used, you should

_____ .

260. If cotton and towels are saturated with solution, what should you do?

_____

261. How long should you process for?

_____

262. What affects the amount of processing time?

a) _____   c) _____

b) _____

263. Describe what the stylist is doing in the illustration below.

_____

264. When processing is completed you should rinse the hair thoroughly, for at least _____ minutes.

a) two

b) three

c) four

d) five

265. What is the best way to towel-blot the hair to be sure to remove excess moisture?

_____

266. If the product requires the application of a pre-neutralizing conditioner when would it be applied?

_____

267. Apply the neutralizer quickly, making sure to pour it around the head.

_____ True

_____ False

268. How long should the neutralizer remain on the hair?

_____

269. After you remove the rods you should rinse the hair thoroughly for five minutes.

_____ True

_____ False

270. Describe the cleanup procedure for this service.

a) _____

b) _____

c) _____

d) _____

e) _____

Safety Precautions

271. It is advisable to apply a hydroxide relaxer on hair that has been previously treated with a thio relaxer.

_____ True

_____ False

272. Do not apply a thio relaxer on hair that has been previously treated with a hydroxide relaxer.

_____ True

_____ False

273. Do not chemically relax hair that has been treated with a metallic dye.

_____ True

_____ False

274. It is advisable to shampoo the client prior to the application of a hydroxide relaxer.

_____ True

_____ False

275. The client's hair and scalp must be completely dry and free from perspiration prior to the application of a hydroxide relaxer.

_____ True

_____ False

276. If any solution accidentally gets into the client's eye, you should

_____ .

277. Do not attempt to remove more than _____ of the natural curl.

a) 20%

b) 40%

c) 60%

d) 80%

278. What can occur if you fail to thoroughly rinse the chemical relaxer from the hair?

_____

279. What can you use to restore the hair and scalp to their normal acidic pH?

_____

280. Why should you use a neutralizing shampoo with a color indicator?

_____

281. Why should you use a conditioner and wide-tooth comb when combing out tangles?

_____

282. It is safe to use hot irons or excessive heat on chemically relaxed hair.

_____ True

_____ False

16

HAIRCOLORING

Date: _____

Rating: _____

Text Pages: 545-602

POINT TO PONDER:

"Nothing is a waste of time if you use the experience wisely."—Auguste Rodin

1. What is one of the most lucrative areas in which a stylist can choose to work?

_____

2. What are some reasons why clients color their hair?

_____

3. How often do clients who have their hair colored usually visit the salon?

_____ a) every four to five weeks
_____ b) every four to six weeks
_____ c) every four to twelve weeks
_____ d) every four to fifteen weeks

CONSULTATION

4. Why is the consultation the most critical part of the color service?

_____

_____

5. Before beginning a haircolor service you will have to determine whether your clients have any

_____ or _____ to the mixture.

6. What does the U.S. Federal Food, Drug, and Cosmetic Act prescribe to identify an allergy in a client?

_____

7. What is another name for a patch test?

   _____

8. Is a patch test required for each and every color service, regardless of the color category?

   _____

9. When is the patch test given?

   _____ a) just before the service
   _____ b) 24 to 48 hours prior to application
   _____ c) 72 to 96 hours after an application
   _____ d) just after the application

10. To perform the patch test, it is permissible to use leftover haircolor from another client's service as long as it is a different color than the client will be receiving.

    _____ True

    _____ False

11. It is advisable to use the same shade of color even if it is a different manufacturer's brand from the one that will actually be used during the color service.

    _____ True

    _____ False

12. Where is the best place to apply the tint for the patch test?

    _____

13. How should the area selected be prepared to receive the tint?

    _____

14. Tint used for a patch test is not mixed with developer prior to being put on the client's skin.

    _____ True

    _____ False

15. Identify the action illustrated below.

_____

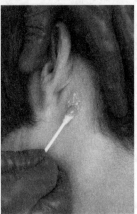

16. The tint should remain undisturbed on the test site for

_____ a) 24 minutes
_____ b) 2 hours
_____ c) 12 hours
_____ d) 24 hours

17. How do you know if it is safe to proceed with the color service?

_____

18. A/an _____ skin test will show no sign of inflammation and indicates that the color

may be safely applied.

   a) positive

   b) negative

   c) neutral

   d) advanced

19. A/an _____ skin test will show redness and a slight rash or welt.

   a) positive

   b) negative

   c) neutral

   d) advanced

HAIRCOLOR APPLICATION PROCEDURES

20. To ensure successful results when performing haircoloring services, the colorist may create a system that is easy and comfortable for her to follow.

    _____ True

    _____ False

21. A clearly defined system makes for the greatest _____ and the safest and most

    _____ results.

22. What is a preliminary strand test?

    _____

    _____

23. When is the strand test performed?

    _____

24. List the implements and materials you will need to perform the preliminary strand test

    a) _____   h) _____

    b) _____   i) _____

    c) _____   j) _____

    d) _____   k) _____

    e) _____   l) _____

    f) _____   m) _____

    g) _____

25. During the client consultation and before the strand test, you must perform a _____

    analysis.

26. After draping the client, part off a _____ square strand of hair in the lower crown and, using plastic clips, fasten other hair out of the way.

    a) $\frac{1}{4}''$

    b) $\frac{1}{2}''$

    c) $\frac{3}{4}''$

    d) $1''$

27. How should you apply the color formula to this section of hair?

_____

28. What application method should be used for the strand test?

_____

29. Check the development at _____ -minute intervals until the desired color has been achieved.

   a) 1

   b) 3

   c) five

   d) 7

30. Once you believe that satisfactory color has developed what should you do?

_____

_____

_____

31. Seeing the results of this strand test will allow you to _____ the formula, the timing, or

   the application method as necessary before you proceed with the color service.

32. In what forms is temporary color available?

_____

33. List all the implements and materials needed for a temporary haircolor application.

   a) _____   f) _____

   b) _____   g) _____

   c) _____   h) _____

   d) _____   i) _____

   e) _____   j) _____

34. Why should you perform a client consultation before a temporary haircolor application?

_____

35. Ask the client to remove any _____ , and keep it in a safe place.

36. How should you drape the client?

    _____

37. Describe the steps in draping a client for a haircolor service.

    a) _____

    _____

    b) _____

    _____

    c) _____

    _____

    d) _____

    _____

38. Temporary color is applied to dry hair.

    _____ True

    _____ False

39. Where is the temporary color applied?

    _____ a) under a hood dryer
    _____ b) at the shampoo bowl
    _____ c) at your station
    _____ d) in the dispensary

40. List the steps in applying temporary color.

    a) _____

    b) _____

    c) _____

    d) _____

    e) _____

    f) _____

41. How should you clean up after a temporary color application?

a) _____

b) _____

c) _____

d) _____

e) _____

42. _____ colors lack the strong oxidizers necessary to lift color; they deposit color and do no substantial lifting.

43. What is the key rule to remember when selecting a semipermanent color?

_____

44. What determines how well a semipermanent product "takes?"

_____

45. Why might semipermanent color build up on the hair ends?

_____

46. A strand test before a semipermanent color application will determine your formula and processing time before each service.

_____ True

_____ False

47. What implements and materials are needed for a semipermanent haircolor application?

a) _____   i) _____

b) _____   j) _____

c) _____   k) _____

d) _____   l) _____

e) _____   m) _____

f) _____   n) _____

g) _____   o) _____

h) _____

48. Before the application of semipermanent color you should perform a preliminary patch test _____ hours before the service.

49. In preparation for the service you will want to do the following.

a) _____

b) _____

c) _____

d) _____

e) _____

f) _____

50. The client's hair should always be shampooed with a mild shampoo and towel-dried before color is applied.

_____ True

_____ False

51. Since there is no developer used, you are not required to wear protective gloves.

_____ True

_____ False

52. Semipermanent color is applied to the scalp and root area first and then worked up to the midshaft.

_____ True

_____ False

53. How is semipermanent color applied?

_____

54. Once the color is applied you should

_____ a) put the client under the dryer
_____ b) rinse the color immediately
_____ c) pile the hair loosely on top of the head
_____ d) cover the head with a moist towel

55. All semipermanent hair colors require the use of a plastic cap.

_____ True

_____ False

56. What should you use as a guide for the processing time?

   _____

57. When the color has developed, shampoo the hair with a mild shampoo.

   _____ True

   _____ False

58. How will you clean up after the service?

   a) _____

   b) _____

   c) _____

59. The application procedure for a _____ haircolor is similar to that of a

   semipermanent color, since neither color alters the hair's natural melanin or produces lift.

60. Why does gray hair present special challenges when formulating demipermanent haircolor?

   _____

   _____

61. It is usually not advisable to color gray hair _____ , since natural hair

   color has different depths and tonalities that give it the added life that gray hair is lacking.

   a) One uneven shade

   b) Two uneven shades

   c) One even shade

   d) Two even shades

62. How does porosity affect demipermanent haircolor?

   _____

63. Permanent haircolor applications are classified as either _____ process or_____

   process.

64. _____ haircoloring is a process that lightens and colors the hair in a single

   application.

65. Give two examples of single-process coloring: _____ and

_____ .

66. What is a virgin application?

_____

67. Prelightening or presoftening is required for a virgin application.

_____ True

_____ False

68. Single-process tints usually contain a _____ , a _____ , an

_____ , and an _____ to activate the

added peroxide.

69. Most color is formulated to be used with _____ volume peroxide.

   a) 5

   b) 10

   c) 15

   d) 20

70. What happens when other volumes of peroxide are used?

_____

71. _____ is a technique requiring two separate procedures in which the

hair is prelightened before the depositing color is applied.

72. Why is double-process color desirable?

_____

_____

73. List the four basic questions that must always be asked when formulating a haircolor.

a) _____

b) _____

c) _____

d) _____

74. What determines the lifting ability of a haircolor?

_____

75. Why should you always remember to formulate with both lift and deposit in mind?

_____

76. If you use a higher lifting formula, what should you take into account?

_____

_____

77. What other component will also influence the lift and deposit?

_____

78. What determines your method of mixing permanent colors?

_____

79. How is permanent color applied?

_____

80. If using an applicator bottle, how large should it be?

_____

_____

81. How should color be mixed with a 1:1 ratio?

_____

_____

82. How should color be mixed with a 2:1 ratio?

_____

83. What type of color normally uses a 2:1 ratio?

_____

84. If using a brush and bowl, what type of bowl should be used?

_____

85. How is color mixed in the bowl?

_____

_____

86. How is the formula mixed in the color bowl?

_____

87. What will the mixture look like when completely blended?

_____

88. What additional implements and materials will you need for a single-process color for virgin hair?

a) _____

b) _____

c) _____

89. A patch test is not necessary for permanent hair color.

_____ True

_____ False

90. Hair should not be shampooed prior to putting the permanent color on.

_____ True

_____ False

91. How many sections should the hair be parted into?

_____ a) two
_____ b) three
_____ c) four
_____ d) five

92. You should prepare the tint formula for either bottle or brush application

_____ a) before you section the hair
_____ b) after you section the hair
_____ c) before you drape the client
_____ d) after you sanitize the tint brush

93. Where should you begin applying color?

_____

_____

94. When applying color part off a _____ subsection with the applicator.

a) $\frac{1}{8}''$

b) $\frac{1}{4}''$

c) $\frac{1}{2}''$

d) 1"

95. Lift the subsection and apply color to the _____ area.

96. Be sure to stay at least _____ from the scalp, and do not go through the porous ends.

a) $\frac{1}{8}''$

b) $\frac{1}{4}''$

c) $\frac{1}{2}''$

d) 1"

97. How long should you process the color?

_____

98. Identify the action illustrated below.

_____

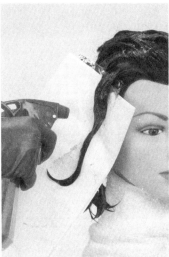

99. After the hair in the midshaft is processed, where should you apply color?

_____

100. Once completely processed, how should the color be removed?

_____

101. How should you remove any stains around the hairline?

_____

102. How do you finish the service?

_____

103. As the hair grows, you will need to _____ it to keep it looking attractive and to avoid a

two-toned effect.

104. What is the difference between a retouch application and the virgin single-process procedure?

_____

105. Overlapping tint can cause _____ and can create a line of _____ .

106. What is a line of demarcation?

_____

107. What should be applied to the ends to freshen and blend them with the new color?

    _____

108. With what should you dilute the remaining tint mixture?

    _____

109. When should you prelighten hair?

    _____

110. Why is it more efficient to use a double-process application?

    _____

    _____

111. How is prelightener applied?

    _____

112. Once the prelightening has reached the desired shade, the hair is lightly _____ ,

    _____ , and _____ .

113. Before applying the new color what type of test should be done?

    _____ a) porosity
    _____ b) elasticity
    _____ c) strand
    _____ d) pulling

LIGHTENING TECHNIQUES

114. Name the three forms of lighteners.

    a) _____
    b) _____
    c) _____

115. Match the following types of lighteners with where they are applied.

    _____ 1. oil lightener   A. on-the-scalp
    _____ 2. powder lightener   B. on-the-scalp
    _____ 3. cream lightener   C. off-the scalp

116. Why are cream and oil lighteners the most popular type of lighteners?

_____

117. _____ lighteners are the mildest type, appropriate when only one or two levels of

color lift are desired.

118. _____ lighteners are strong enough to do blonding, but gentle enough to be used

on the scalp.

119. Cream lighteners may be mixed with _____ in the form of dry crystals.

120. An _____ is an oxidizer added to hydrogen peroxide to increase its chemical action

or its lifting power.

121. How many activators can be used for on-the-scalp applications?

_____

122. How many activators can be used for off-the-scalp applications?

_____

123. Powder lightener is a _____, _____ lightener in powdered form.

124. Can powder lightener be used to do blonding?

_____

125. How do powder lighteners work?

_____

126. Why should powder lighteners *not* be used for retouch services?

_____

127. What effect does the hair's natural melanin have on processing time?

_____

_____

128 What effect does the hair's porosity have on processing time?

_____

_____

129. What effect does the hair's natural tone have on processing time?

_____

_____

130. _____ blondes are especially difficult to achieve because the melanin must be diffused

sufficiently to alter both the level and tone of the hair.

131. The _____ of the product also affects the speed and amount of lightening because

the stronger lighteners attain the pale shades in the fastest time.

132. What effect does heat have on lightening?

_____

133. If using heat in the lightening process, what must be carefully observed?

_____

_____

134. What can happen if the hair is too light before the toner is applied?

_____

135. Perform a preliminary _____ prior to lightening to determine the process time, the

condition of the hair after lightening, and the end results.

136. If the test shows the hair is not light enough, you should _____

_____.

137. If the hair strand is too light, you should _____

_____.

138. List all of the implements and materials you will need for lightening virgin hair.

a) _____   i) _____

b) _____   j) _____

c) _____   k) _____

d) _____   l) _____

e) _____   m) _____

f) _____   n) _____

g) _____   o) _____

h) _____

139. How many sections should the hair be divided into?

_____

140. Should the hair be wet or dry for a lightening service?_____

141. Apply a _____ around the hairline and over the ears.

142. It isn't necessary to wear protective gloves for a lightening procedure.

_____ True

_____ False

143. When should you prepare the lightening formula?

_____ a) one hour before the procedure
_____ b) after draping the client
_____ c) immediately before using it
_____ d) after toner is applied

144. What can you place at the scalp area along the parts to prevent the lightener from touching the base of the hair?

_____

145. To apply the lightener, you should begin the application where the hair seems_____

or_____ , usually at the back of the head.

146. What size partings should be used to apply the lightener?

_____ a) ⅛"

_____ b) ¼"

_____ c) ½"

_____ d) 1"

147. Start

_____ a) ¹⁄₁₆"

_____ b) ⅛"

_____ c) ¼"

_____ d) ½"

148. Lightener should be applied to the top of the strand in quick movements.

_____ True

_____ False

149. Why is a strip of cotton placed between sections?

_____

150. Once all of the lightener is applied, double check the application and _____ lightener

if necessary.

151. Comb the lightener through the hair to make sure it is well covered.

_____ True

_____ False

152. Keep the lightener moist during development by reapplying as the mixture dries on the hair.

_____ True

_____ False

153. Check for lightening action about _____ minutes before the time indicated by the preliminary

strand test.

_____ a) five

_____ b) 8

_____ c) 12

_____ d) 15

154. When checking the strand, spray it with _____ and remove the lightener with a damp towel.

    a) lightener

    b) peroxide

    c) water

    d) activator

155. If the strand is not light enough, _____

    _____ .

156. Once the midshaft is properly processed, remove the cotton from the scalp area and apply the lightener

    to the hair near the scalp with a _____ parting.

    a) $^{1}/_{16}$"

    b) $^{1}/_{8}$"

    c) $^{1}/_{4}$"

    d) $^{1}/_{2}$"

157. When applying lightener to the scalp area, simply re-wet the lightener you mixed earlier.

    _____ True

    _____ False

158. Rinse the hair thoroughly with _____ water.

    a) freezing

    b) cool

    c) tepid

    d) hot

159. Where should you place your hands while shampooing and conditioning the hair?

    _____

160. How do you neutralize the alkalinity of the hair?

_____

161. After the lightener is removed, you may apply toner to freshly shampooed hair.

_____ True

_____ False

162. After the hair is dried you will want to examine the:

a) _____

b) _____

163. Once you've checked the scalp and condition of the hair, you may proceed with a _____

application if desired.

164. As the lightened hair grows, dark new growth or _____ will become very obvious,

and it will need to be lightened.

165. The procedure for a lightener retouch is the same as that for lightening a virgin head of hair, except that

the mixture is applied only to the _____.

166. What type of lightener is generally used for a lightener retouch because its consistency helps prevent
overlapping of previously lightened hair?

_____

167. _____ are used primarily on prelightened hair to achieve pale, delicate colors.

168. Toners do not require a double-process application.

_____ True

_____ False

169. The first step of the double-process procedure is to _____ and the second step

is to _____.

170. How many stages of decolorization will the hair go through? _____

171. The color that is left in the hair after decolorization is known as its _____ .

172. Why is it is essential that you achieve the correct foundation for proper toner development?

_____

173. How will you know what foundation you need for the toner color selected?

_____

_____

174. As a general rule, the paler the color you are seeking, the _____ the foundation you will need.

 a) darker

 b) brighter

 c) dimmer

 d) lighter

175. How does overlightened hair behave when toner is applied?

_____

176. How does underlightened hair behave when toner is applied?

_____

177. It is not advisable to prelighten past the _____ stage.

178. What may occur if you prelighten past the pale yellow stage?

_____

_____

179. You will need to administer a patch test for allergies or other sensitivities to toners 24 hours before the application.

 _____ True

 _____ False

180. To save time, you may do a _____ on the same day as the patch test.

181. You can proceed with the application only if the patch test results are _____ and

the hair is in good condition.

182. Wearing gloves throughout the application of toner is not necessary.

_____ True

_____ False

183. What factors will determine whether you get good results from the toner application?

_____

185. All toners are mixed with peroxide.

_____ True

_____ False

185. List all of the implements and materials you need for toner application.

a) _____   i) _____

b) _____   j) _____

c) _____   k) _____

d) _____   l) _____

e) _____   m) _____

f) _____   n) _____

g) _____   o) _____

h) _____

186. Before applying toner, the hair must be _____.

187. Once the desired toner shade is selected, apply _____ around the hairline

and over the ears.

188. What is an oxidative toner?

_____

189. If using an oxidative toner, what type of container should you use to mix the toner and the developer in?

_____

190. How many sections should the hair be divided into?

_____ a) two
_____ b) three
_____ c) four
_____ d) five

190. Where should the toner application begin?

_____

191. Part off _____ partings and apply the toner from the scalp up to, but not including, the porous ends.

a) $\frac{1}{8}''$

b) $\frac{1}{4}''$

c) $\frac{1}{2}''$

d) 1″

192. Once you have taken a strand test and it indicates proper color development, what should you do?

_____

193. Once the entire head is covered in toner, how should you treat the hair?

_____

_____

194. How should you remove the toner?

_____

195. Why should you apply conditioner to the toned hair?

_____

196. Why should you be careful not to stretch toned hair?

_____

SPECIAL EFFECTS HAIRCOLORING

197. Special effects haircoloring is any technique that involves partial_____ or _____.

198. Describe one way to create special effects in the hair.

_____

199. Highlighting involves coloring some of the hair strands_____ than the natural color to

add the illusion of sheen and depth.

200. Highlights generally contrast strongly with the natural hair color.

_____ True

_____ False

201. Light colors cause an area to:

a) _____

b) _____

c) _____

202. Reverse highlighting, or _____ , is the technique of coloring strands of hair darker

than the natural color.

203. Contrasting dark areas_____.

204. The three most frequently used techniques for achieving highlights are.

a) _____   c) _____

b) _____

205. The cap technique involves:_____

_____.

206. What determines the degree of highlighting or lowlighting you can achieve?

_____

207. When only a small number of strands are pulled through, the result will be a _____ look.

208. When a greater number of strands are pulled through, a more _____ effect is achieved.

209. For highlighting, the hair is usually lightened with a _____.

210. How is the lightener removed from the cap?

_____

211. How should toner be applied to the highlighted hair?

_____

212. The foil technique involves coloring selected strands of hair by _____

_____

_____

213. When would you apply permanent haircolor to the strands instead of lightening products?

_____

214. How can you practice the foil technique before actually foiling a head?

_____

215. Describe a slicing.

_____

_____

216. Describe weaving.

_____

_____

217. List the different patterns in which foil can be placed in the hair.

a) _____   c) _____

b) _____   d) _____

218. Each wrapping pattern is used to _____.

219. List all of the implements and materials you need for a special effects haircoloring with foil.

a) _____   g) _____

b) _____   h) _____

c) _____   i) _____

d) _____   j) _____

e) _____   k) _____

f) _____

220. A patch test is not necessary for a highlighting service.

_____ True

_____ False

221. Where on the head should you begin foiling?

_____

222. Once the hair is sliced out you should _____.

223. Holding the hair _____, brush on the lightener, from the upper edge of the foil to the hair ends.

a) limp

b) sideways

c) upside down

d) taut

224. How should you enclose the hair in the foil?

_____

_____

225. Where should the foil be put to keep it out of the way?

_____

226. How much space should be left between foils?

_____

227. Once the entire section is complete you can _____ .

228. How should hair around the face be sliced?

_____

229. Once the lightener in the foils has processed according to the strand test, how are the foils removed?

   _____ a) one section at a time
   _____ b) half of the head at a time
   _____ c) one at a time
   _____ d) back section first and then the front section

230. Where should the foils be removed?

   _____ a) at the station
   _____ b) in the dispensary
   _____ c) in the rest room
   _____ d) at the shampoo bowl

231. Why should you rinse the hair immediately?

_____

232. After the color is removed from the hair what may you decide to apply?

_____

233. The balayage or free-form technique involves the painting of a lightener directly onto

_____ .

234. What type of lightener is generally used for the balayage technique? _____

235. What tool is used to apply the lightener? _____

236. The effects of the balayage technique are _____ and are used to draw attention

to the surface of the hair.

   a) extremely noticeable

   b) brilliantly bright

   c) deep and dark

   d) extremely subtle

237. If you want to achieve a cool tonality in prelightened hair you will want to use a toner to _____

_____ .

238. When using a toner on highlighted hair, it is important to consider _____

_____ .

239. An _____ toner would impart color to the highlighted strands, but it might also affect

the natural, or pigmented, hair, causing a slight amount of lift.

240. The result of an oxidative toner may be _____

_____ .

241. To avoid affecting untreated hair, list the choices you might make instead of an oxidative toner:

a) _____   c) _____

b) _____

242. What are the ingredients in highlighting shampoo tints?

a) _____   c) _____

b) _____

243. What type of effect do highlighting shampoo tints give?

_____

244. What do they actually do?

_____

245. No patch test is required for a highlighting shampoo tint service.

_____ True

_____ False

246. Highlighting shampoos are a mixture of _____ and _____ .

247. What effect do highlighting shampoos impart?

_____

248. A patch test is required for a highlighting shampoo service.

_____ True

_____ False

249. Clients who have been either tinting or lightening and who want to return to their natural shade need a

process called a _____.

250. What are some of the things that can alter the hair color?

_____

251. What effect does porous hair have on the tint-back procedure?

_____

_____

252. List two options for a client returning to her natural color after wearing it lighter for any length of time.

a) _____

b) _____

253. The key to a successful tint back to natural color hair may be the use of a _____ to even

out the porosity and to achieve color correction.

254. What is a soap cap and why is it useful?

_____

_____

_____

255. A quick soap cap will break the _____.

17

HISTOLOGY OF THE SKIN

See Milady's Standard Cosmetology Theory Workbook

18

HAIR REMOVAL

Date: _____

Rating: _____

Text Pages: 631-651

POINT TO PONDER:

"It takes a lot of time to get experience, and once you have it you ought to go on using it."—Benjamin M. Duggar

1. The scientific term for the growth of an unusual amount of hair on parts of the body normally bearing only downy hair, such as the faces of women or the backs of men, is _____ .

2. Where do women most want to remove unwanted hair?

   _____

3. Where do men most want to remove unwanted hair?

   _____

4. Name the two major types of hair removal in use today.

   a) _____

   b) _____

5. Salon techniques are generally considered permanent.

   _____ True

   _____ False

CLIENT CONSULTATION

6. What questions should a client be asked prior to giving a hair removal service?

   a) _____

   b) _____

7. After their first hair removal service, how often should you ask the client these questions?

_____ a) every visit

_____ b) every other visit

_____ c) every year

_____ d) every other year

8. What is a contraindication?

_____

_____

9. What are the contraindications for hair removal services?

a) _____

b) _____

c) _____

d) _____

e) _____

f) _____

g) _____

10. Clients using the following medications should also not receive hair removal treatments.

a) _____

b) _____

c) _____

d) _____

PERMANENT HAIR REMOVAL

11. Name the methods of permanent hair removal.

a) _____

b) _____

c) _____

12. The removal of hair by means of an electric current that destroys the root of the hair is called

    _____ .

13. In electrolysis how is the current applied?

    _____

14. Who can perform electrolysis?

    _____

15. What is photo-epilation?

    _____

16. Does this treatment use needles?

    _____

17. Who can administer photo-epiliation?

    _____

18. _____ are a new method for the rapid, gentle removal of unwanted hair.

19. In laser hair removal, a laser beam is _____ , impairing the hair follicles.

20. Laser is most effective when used on follicles in the active growing phase, called _____ .

21. What type of hair responds best to laser treatment?

    _____

22. Is laser hair removal permanent?

    _____

23. Who can perform laser hair removal?

    _____

TEMPORARY METHODS OF HAIR REMOVAL

24. Name the methods of temporary hair removal:

a) _____ e) _____

b) _____ f) _____

c) _____ g) _____

d) _____

25. What is the most common form of temporary hair removal?

_____

26. When is shaving recommended for women?

_____

27. A shaving cream or lotion is applied _____ shaving.

a) before

b) during

c) after

d) while

28. What effects can result from shaving?

_____

29. What can be done help to reduce any irritation?

_____

30. Where should you performing a shaving service?

_____

31. List the implements and tools needed to perform a shaving service.

    a) _____ d) _____

    b) _____ e) _____

    c) _____ f) _____

32. How should you prepare for giving a shaving service?

    a) _____

    b) _____

    c) _____

33. How should you drape a client for this service?

    _____

    _____

34. How should you prepare the clients face for shaving?

    _____

    _____

35. If your client has sensitive or rosacea skin, what temperature should the towel be?

    _____

36. From where should you be administering shaving cream and what should you use to apply it to the face?

    _____

37. To begin shaving you should stretch the skin tautly with one hand, use the other to stroke the razor in the direction of the hair growth.

    _____ True

    _____ False

38. Where should you begin shaving?

    _____

    _____

39. After the jawline is shaved, where should you go next?

    _____

40. While completing the shave, you must not rinse the razor.

    _____ True

    _____ False

41. After the face has been shaved, cleanse it with another _____, damp towel, depending

    on the skin type.

42. After the shave apply:

    _____ a) hydrogen peroxide
    _____ b) alcohol
    _____ c) antiseptic
    _____ d) after-shave lotion

43. Used towels and cape may be used on the next client.

    _____ True

    _____ False

44. Describe the rest of the steps in cleaning up after a shaving service.

    a) _____

    b) _____

    c) _____

45. _____ is commonly used to shape the eyebrows and can also be used to remove undesirable

    hairs from around the mouth and chin.

46. When is eyebrow arching commonly done?

    _____

47. Why are correctly shaped eyebrows important?

    _____

48. The natural arch of the eyebrow follows the _____, or the curved line of the eye socket.

49. From where should hair be removed to give a clean and attractive appearance?

    _____

50. List all of the implements and materials needed to perform a tweezing service.

    a) _____

    b) _____

    c) _____

    d) _____

    e) _____

    f) _____

    g) _____

    h) _____

    i) _____

51. How should you and your client prepare for an eyebrow tweezing service?

    a) _____

    b) _____

    c) _____

    d) _____

52. It is acceptable to begin tweezing the eyebrow without removing eye makeup.

    _____ True

    _____ False

53. _____ the eyebrows to remove any powder or scaliness.

    a) wax

    b) tweeze

    c) brush

    d) remove

54. Why would you saturate two pledgets of cotton or a towel with warm water and place over the eyebrows?

_____

55. Use a _____ on a cotton ball prior to tweezing.

   a) strong alcohol

   b) strong antiseptic

   c) mild peroxide

   d) mild antiseptic

56. From where will you be tweezing hair?

_____

57. How should you hold the skin when tweezing?

_____

58. How many hairs should be tweezed at once?

_____

59. To avoid infection you should _____

_____

60. After tweezing is completed, sponge the eyebrows and surrounding skin with _____ to contract the skin.

61. The final step of the tweezing service is to _____.

62. Once completed and if the eyebrow tweezing is part of a makeup service, you can continue the makeup procedure.

   _____ True

   _____ False

63. If no more services are to be performed, how should you clean up after a tweezing service?

    a) _____

    b) _____

    c) _____

    d) _____

64. The eyebrows should be treated about once a:

    _____ a) day
    _____ b) week
    _____ c) month
    _____ d) year

65. How do electronically charged tweezers work?

    _____

    _____

66. How do you use electronic tweezers?

    _____

    _____

67. It is helpful to _____ the area first in order to increase efficiency.

68. Electronic tweezers are a method of permanent hair removal.

    _____ True

    _____ False

69. A _____ is a substance, usually a caustic alkali preparation, used for the temporary removal of superfluous hair by dissolving it at the skin level.

70. What happens to the hair during the application time of a depilatory?

    _____

71. Where are depilatories most commonly used?

    _____ a) hair salon
    _____ b) at home
    _____ c) nail salon
    _____ d) luxury spa

72. If a client requests a chemical depilatory, you should perform a _____ to determine whether the individual is sensitive to the action of the depilatory.

73. A/an _____ removes the hair by pulling it out of the follicle.

74. _____ is a commonly used epilator, applied in either hot or cold form as recommended by the manufacturer.

75. Why does it take between four to six weeks to perform another waxing service?

    _____

76. Where can wax be applied on the body?

    _____

    _____

77. Do men use waxing service?

    _____

78. To be effective, how long should the hair be for a waxing service?

    _____

79. Before beginning a wax treatment, be sure to complete a _____ and have the client sign a _____ .

80. Why should you wear disposable gloves?

    _____

81. List the equipment, implements, and materials needed to perform an eyebrow waxing.

a) _____   h) _____

b) _____   i) _____

c) _____   j) _____

d) _____   k) _____

e) _____   l) _____

f) _____   m) _____

g) _____   n) _____

82. Describe how you prepare yourself and your client for an eyebrow waxing.

a) _____

b) _____

c) _____

d) _____

e) _____

f) _____

83. What is the procedure for an eyebrow wax?

a) _____

b) _____

c) _____

d) _____
   _____

e) _____
   _____

f) _____
   _____

g) _____

h) _____

i) _____

j) _____

84. Describe how to clean up after the service is completed.

    a) _____

    b) _____

    c) _____

       _____

    d) _____

85. How should you prepare to give a full body wax?

    a) _____

    b) _____

    c) _____

    d) _____

    e) _____

86. If bikini waxing, offer the client disposable _____ or a _____ .

87. If waxing the underarms, have the client remove her bra and put on a _____ .

88. What should the client wear when waxing the legs?

    _____

89. Thoroughly cleanse the area to be waxed with a _____ and dry.

90. Before you begin, apply a light covering of _____ to the area to be waxed.

    a) water

    b) powder

    c) astringent

    d) alcohol

91. You must always test the temperature and consistency of the heated wax by applying a small drop to your wrist.

_____ True
_____ False

92. How should you apply the wax to the area you desire to treat?

_____

_____

93. If wax lands in an area you do not wish to treat, what should you do?

_____

94. How do you take the wax off?

_____

_____

_____

95. Why should you lightly massage the treated area?

_____

96. After you have completed the entire area to be waxed you should _____

_____

_____ .

97. How should you clean up after a full body wax?

a) _____

b) _____

c) _____

d) _____

e) _____

f) _____

98. Should you apply wax over warts, moles, abrasions, or irritated or inflamed skin?

    _____

99. If redness and swelling occur on sensitive skin what should be done?

    _____

100. _____ is a temporary hair removal method that involves the manipulation of cotton thread, which is twisted and rolled along the surface of the skin, entwining the hair in the thread and lifting it from the follicle.

101. _____, another epilator treatment, involves the use of a thick, sugar-based paste and is especially appropriate for more sensitive skin types.

102. After a sugaring procedure, any residue can be dissolved with _____.

19

FACIALS

Date: _____

Rating:_____

Text Pages: 653-693

POINT TO PONDER:

"A thought may be very commendable as a thought, but I value it chiefly as a window through which I can obtain insight on the thinker."—Alexander Smith

1. What service do clients often consider their favorite part of a salon visit?

   _____

2. If performed correctly and professionally, the facial can serve as an oasis in a busy day, leaving the client

   feeling _____ .

3. A facial can _____

   _____ .

4. Your work will be particularly valuable to many of your clients for who skin problems cause _____

   _____ .

5. All massage treatments combine basic movements or manipulations which are applied to the

   _____ in a certain way to achieve a certain end.

6. The impact of a massage treatment depends on:

   a) _____

   b) _____

   c) _____

7. The direction of movement always starts at the origin of the muscle.

   _____ True

   _____ False

8. The movement goes from the insertion toward the _____ , which is the fixed attachment of one end of the muscle to a bone or tissue.

9. Massaging a muscle in the wrong direction could result in

_____ .

10. _____ is a light, continuous stroking movement applied with the fingers or the palms in a slow, rhythmic manner.

11. How much pressure is used in effleurage?

_____ a) extreme

_____ b) moderate

_____ c) light

_____ d) none

12. Where is effleurage most frequently used?

_____

13. What effects does effleurage have?

_____

14. Effleurage should be used in the middle of every massage.

_____ True

_____ False

15. When performing effleurage, how should you hold your hand?

_____

_____

_____

16. _____ is a kneading movement performed by lifting, squeezing, and pressing the tissue with a light, firm pressure.

17. What kind of massage does petrissage offer?

_____

18. Petrissage is most often used on which parts of the body?

_____

19. Done lightly, petrissage may also be used on the cheeks with_____.

20. The pressure should be _____.

21. When grasping and releasing fleshy areas, the movements must be _____, never jerky.

22. _____ is a form of petrissage in which the tissue is grasped, gently lifted, and

spread out, used mainly for massaging the arms.

23. How do you perform fulling?

_____

_____

24. _____ is a deep rubbing movement in which you apply pressure on the skin with

your fingers or palm while moving it over an underlying structure.

25. Friction can benefit the _____.

26. Circular friction movements are usually used on the _____.

27. When friction is applied in light circular movements, the practitioner is usually working on the

_____.

28. _____ , _____ , and _____ are variations of friction and are

used principally to massage the arms and legs.

29. _____ is accomplished by grasping the flesh firmly in one hand and moving the

hand up and down along the bone while the other hand keeps the arm or leg in a steady position.

30. _____ is accomplished when the tissues are pressed and twisted using a fast back-and-forth movement.

31. _____ is a vigorous movement in which the hands, placed a little distance apart on both sides of the client's arm or leg and working downward, apply a twisting motion against the bones in the opposite direction.

32. _____, or _____, consists of short, quick tapping, slapping, and hacking movements.

33. Petrissage is the most stimulating and should be applied with care and discretion.

    _____ True

    _____ False

34. Tapotement movements are used for what effect?

    _____

35. How are tapotement movements used in facial massage?

    _____

    _____

36. _____ is a chopping movement performed with the edges of the hands.

37. Describe how hacking is performed.

    _____

38. Where are hacking and slapping movements used?

    _____

39. _____ is a rapid shaking of the body part while the balls of the fingertips are pressed firmly on the point of application.

40. How is vibration performed?

    _____

41. Vibration is a highly stimulating movement.

    _____ True

    _____ False

42. Vibration should be applied at the end of the massage.

    _____ True

    _____ False

43. _____ in combination with other classical massage movements can also be produced by the use of a mechanical vibrator to stimulate blood circulation and increase muscle tone in muscles of the body.

44. _____ are restricted to the massage of the arm, hand and foot.

45. Joint movements are always applied with resistance.

    _____ True

    _____ False

46. Every muscle has a _____, which is a point on the skin over the muscle where pressure or stimulation will cause contraction of that muscle.

47. In order to obtain the maximum benefits from a facial massage, you must consider the motor points that affect the _____.

48. The location of motor points is the same from person to person.

    _____ True

    _____ False

49. _____ is achieved through light but firm, slow, rhythmic movements, or very slow, light hand vibrations over the motor points for a short time.

50. The immediate effects of massage on the skin are increases in:

    a) _____   c) _____

    b) _____   d) _____

51. List the benefits a client may experience by obtaining proper facial and scalp massage.

   a) _____

   b) _____

   c) _____

   d) _____

   e) _____

   f) _____

   g) _____

52. What things should be considered when determining the frequency of facial or scalp massage?

   a) _____   c) _____

   b) _____

53. Normal skin or scalp can be kept in excellent condition with the help of a _____ massage, accompanied by proper home care.

   a) hourly

   b) daily

   c) weekly

   d) monthly

54. To obtain maximum relation what things should you keep in mind about how you are performing facial manipulations?

   _____

55. How should you remove your hands from the client's face once you have started the facial massage?

   _____

56. Why are massage movements generally directed toward the origin of a muscle?

   _____

57. Identify each of the following illustrations by matching it with its description.

_____ 1. chin movement

_____ 2. lower cheeks movement

_____ 3. mouth, nose, and cheek movements

_____ 4. linear movement over the forehead

_____ 5. circular movement over the forehead

_____ 6. crisscross movement

_____ 7. stroking movement

_____ 8. brow and eye movement

_____ 9. nose and upper cheek movement

_____ 10. mouth and nose movement

_____ 11. lip and chin movement

_____ 12. optional lip movement

_____ 13. lifting movement of the cheeks

_____ 14. rotary movement of the cheeks

_____ 15. light tapping movement

_____ 16. stroking movement of the neck

_____ 17. circular movement over the neck and chest

A.

B.

C.

D.

E.

F.

G.

H.

I.

j.

K.

L.

M.

N.

O.

P.

Q.

ELECTROTHERAPY AND LIGHT THERAPY

58. The first step in the disincrustation process is to

    _____ .

59. The client holds the passive electrode in his/her _____ hand or you may place the

    wet pad on a comfortable spot on the _____ side of the body.

60. The active electrode should be wrapped in _____ .

61. When you switch on the galvanic machine, check for _____ polarity on the active

    electrode.

    a) positive

    b) negative

    c) high

    d) low

62. Where should you place the active electrode?

    _____

63. You should place the active electrode on the clients face and quickly turn up the intensity of the current.

    _____ True

    _____ False

64. As soon as your client feels a tingling sensation you can _____

    and _____ .

65. To begin the treatment, move the electrode slowly over the oily areas of the face for _____

    minutes.

66. When the treatment is completed, _____

    before breaking contact with the client.

    a) quickly turn down the intensity of the current

    b) slowly turn down the intensity of the current

    c) quickly turn up the intensity of the current

    d) slowly turn up the intensity of the current

67. _____ electrodes are required to complete a faradic or sinusoidal circuit.

    a) Two

    b) Three

    c) Four

    d) Five

68. The cathode is placed on the _____ of the muscle and the anode on the

    _____ of the muscle.

69. Each muscle should be allowed to contract _____ times before moving on to the next

    muscle.

    a) 1 to 4

    b) 5 to 10

    c) 11 to 15

    d) 16 to 20

70. All treatments given with high-frequency current should start with a _____ intensity and

    _____ increase to the required strength.

71. Name the methods for using the high-frequency current.

a)   _____   b)   _____

72. In the direct surface application what kind of treatment products are applied to the client's face.

_____

73. How is the direct surface application given?

_____

_____

74. When you apply and remove the electrode from the skin, where must you hold your finger and why?

_____

75. For a stronger germicidal effect,_____.

76. How is the indirect application given?

_____

77. In the indirect application, when does the cosmetologist hold the electrode?

_____ a)   all of the time

_____ b)   for one minute

_____ c)   for five minutes

_____ d)   at no time

78. To prevent shock, turn_____ the current only after the client has firmly grasped the electrode.

79. Turn the current _____ before you remove the electrode from the client's hand.

80. The indirect application of high-frequency current stimulates _____ without the irritation that could occur with direct application.

81. This treatment is highly beneficial for _____.

FACIAL TREATMENTS

82. Facial treatments fall under two categories.

a) _____   b) _____

83. A preservative treatment is meant to _____

_____

_____ .

84. A corrective treatment is meant to _____

_____ .

85. Facial treatments help to

    a) _____   d) _____

    b) _____   e) _____

    c) _____

86. To help the client relax during a facial treatment you should speak in a _____

_____ .

87. When clients have questions regarding their facial treatments you should _____

_____ .

88. Facials should be performed in a moderately noisy atmosphere.

    _____ True

    _____ False

89. It is acceptable to clean up the facial room at the end of the day to accommodate a busy schedule of clients.

    _____ True

    _____ False

90. For sanitary reasons, you should remove products from containers with clean fingers.

    _____ True

    _____ False

91. If your hands are cold, warm them before touching the client's face.

    _____ True

    _____ False

92. Keep your nails smooth and short so as not to scratch the client's skin.

_____ True

_____ False

93. List the types of equipment you will need to give a basic facial treatment.

a) _____   d) _____

b) _____   e) _____

c) _____   f) _____

94. List the implements and materials you will need for giving a facial.

a) _____   g) _____

b) _____   h) _____

c) _____   i) _____

d) _____   j) _____

e) _____   k) _____

f) _____   l) _____

95. List all of the products necessary when giving a facial.

a) _____   f) _____

b) _____   g) _____

c) _____   h) _____

d) _____   i) _____

e) _____

96. What are some of the additional things you may need to perform a facial?

a) _____

b) _____

c) _____

97. How should you prepare for your client?

_____

98. To put the client at ease before the service you should _____

_____ .

99. How should the client prepare for the facial?

_____

_____

100. Where should the client change prior to the facial?

_____

101. It is acceptable for the client's bare shoulders to come into contact with the facial chair.

_____ True

_____ False

102. How should you drape a client when they are seated in the facial chair?

_____

_____

_____

103. How should you protect the client's hair during a facial?

_____

_____

104. Give the procedure for draping the head.

a) _____

_____

_____

b) _____

_____

_____

_____

_____

d) _____

_____

_____

105. If a female client is wearing something with straps you should

_____ .

106. To make the client comfortable and to get her at the right height you need to

_____ .

107. Before touching the client's face you should _____ .

108. Before every facial you should _____ .

109. List the steps involved in removing facial makeup on the lips.

a) _____

b) _____

c) _____

110. List the steps involved in removing facial makeup on the eyes.

a) _____

_____

b) _____

_____

c) _____

_____

d) _____

_____

111. When removing eye makeup always do so gently; never rub or stretch the skin, as it is very delicate and thin.

_____ True

_____ False

112. Describe the procedure for applying cleanser to the entire face and neck.

a) _____

_____

_____

b) _____

_____

_____

c) _____

_____

_____

d) _____

_____

_____

e) _____

_____

_____

f) _____

_____

_____

g) _____

_____

_____

113. What should you use to remove the cleanser?

_____

114. When removing cleanser where do you begin?

_____

115. You should try to remove all of the cleanser at one time.

_____ True

_____ False

116. You should begin removing the cleanser on the neck area.

_____ True

_____ False

117. How will you know which products to use on the face next?

_____

_____

118. During a facial when should eyebrow arching be done?

_____

119. During a facial when should exfoliation be done?

_____

120. Why do you steam the face?

_____

_____

121. How do you steam the face?

_____

122. How should you select a massage cream?

_____

123. Describe how to apply the massage cream to the face, neck, shoulders, chest, and back in the same

manner as the _____ was applied.

124. Give the procedure for exposing the face to infrared light.

a) _____

b) _____

c) _____

125. After the massage is completed how should you remove the massage cream?

_____

126. What procedure should be followed for removing massage cream?

_____

127. After massage cream is removed what comes next?

_____

128. When should a treatment mask be applied?

_____

129. What is the proper procedure for applying a treatment mask?

a) _____

_____

b) _____

_____

c) _____

_____

d) _____

_____

e) _____

_____

f) _____

_____

130. After the treatment mask is removed, what should be applied?

_____

131. The last step in the facial is to

_____ .

132. Once the facial is complete and before you begin to clean up you should

_____

_____ .

133. Disposable supplies and materials should be _____ .

134. Open product containers should be

_____.

135. Unused cosmetics and other items should be thrown away.

_____ True

_____ False

136. Where should you place used towels, coverlets, head covers, and other linens?

_____

137. Your workstation should be wiped down.

_____ True

_____ False

138. Your hands should be washed with soap and warm water.

_____ True

_____ False

139. List the special problems that must be considered when you are performing a facial.

a) _____   c) _____

b) _____   d) _____

140. Dry skin is caused by an

_____.

141. The facial for dry skin helps correct this condition and can provide better results if a/an _____

_____ is used.

142. Give the procedure for a facial for dry skin using infrared rays.

a) _____

b) _____

c) _____

d) _____

e) _____

f) _____

g) _____

h) _____

i) _____

j) _____

k) _____

l) _____

m) _____

n) _____

143. List the steps in the procedure for a facial for dry skin using galvanic current.

a) _____

b) _____

c) _____

d) _____

e) _____

f) _____

g) _____

h) _____

i) _____

j) _____

k) _____

l) _____

m) _____

n) _____

o) _____

p) _____

144. When using a high-frequency current during a facial, the client should hold the electrode in his

_____ .

145. During the facial you will give manipulations, using the _____ of applying

high-frequency current, for seven to ten minutes.

146. You may use tapping movements and lift your hands from the client's skin when needed.

_____ True

_____ False

147. After the high-frequency current is applied you should apply two or three _____ towels to the

face and neck.

   a) hot

   b) cold

   c) soft

   d) rough

148. Blackheads are a sign of

_____ a) dry skin

_____ b) oily skin

_____ c) aging skin

_____ d) tired skin

149. Comedones are caused by _____

_____ .

150. Give the procedure for a facial that is beneficial to clients with oily skin.

   a) _____

   b) _____

   c) _____

   d) _____

e) _____

f) _____

g) _____

h) _____

i) _____

j) _____

k) _____

l) _____

m) _____

_____

n) _____

o) _____

p) _____

151. What is the proper method for removing comedones?

_____

_____

_____

152. When removing comedones be sure to use your bare fingers or fingernails.

_____ True

_____ False

153. _____ is a disorder of the sebaceous glands that requires thorough and sometimes

ongoing medical attention.

154. If a client with acne is under medical care, the role of the cosmetologist is to work closely with the client's physician, following the physician's instructions as to the kind and frequency of facial treatments.

_____ True

_____ False

155. When handling skin with acne you will generally be limited to the following measures.

a) _____

b) _____

c) _____

d) _____

156. Because skin with acne contains _____ , you must wear _____

_____ and use _____ materials such as cotton cleansing pads.

157. In addition to the materials used for a basic facial, you will need the following for treating acne.

a) _____   d) _____

b) _____   e) _____

c) _____

158. How should you prepare for an acne treatment?

a) _____

b) _____

c) _____

d) _____

159. Give the steps involved in a facial for a person with acne.

a) _____

_____

b) _____

_____

c) _____

_____

d) _____

_____

e) _____

_____

f) _____

_____

g) _____

_____

h) _____

_____

i) _____

_____

20

FACIAL MAKEUP

Date: _____
Rating:_____
Text Pages: 695-734

POINT TO PONDER:

"The years teach much which the days never know."—Ralph Waldo Emerson

1. Through the use of creative _____ people can be transformed for the special events in their lives such as weddings, and proms.

2. Outside the arena of theater and film, most clients prefer to wear makeup that is _____.

3. The main objective of applying makeup is to emphasize the client's _____ while minimizing those features that are _____.

4. What determines how a client's makeup should be applied?

   _____

5. When applying makeup you must take into consideration the:

   a) _____

   b) _____

   c) _____

   d) _____

   e) _____

6. In a professional setting you will be able to use cosmetics to _____

   _____

7. The client's natural beauty can be enhanced by a blend of: _____, _____,

   and_____

COSMETICS FOR FACIAL MAKEUP

8. What product can be credited with the success of the entire makeup application?

_____ a) lipstick
_____ b) eye pencil
_____ c) foundation
_____ d) blush

9. Picking the perfect foundation depends primarily on _____.

10. When correctly matched and applied, foundation creates an _____ for the rest of the makeup application.

11. What determines the selection of foundation color?

_____

12. Skin tones are generally classified as_____ , _____ , or _____.

13. Which of the following colors is NOT generally associated with warm tones?

_____ a) yellow
_____ b) blue
_____ c) orange
_____ d) red

14. Which of the following colors is NOT generally associated with cool tones?

_____ a) blue
_____ b) green
_____ c) pink
_____ d) yellow

15. Describe a neutral skin tone.

_____

16. Foundation color should always be:

_____ a) lighter than the actual skin tone
_____ b) darker than the actual skin tone
_____ c) matched as closely as possible to the actual skin tone
_____ d) matched as closely as possible to the desired skin tone

17. If foundation color is too light, it will:_____.

18. If foundation color is too dark, it will:_____.

19. To determine the correct foundation color for your client, apply a stripe of color to clean skin on the:

   _____ a) arm
   _____ b) hand
   _____ c) jawline
   _____ d) ear

20. You will know you have the correct color if it _____ on the skin.

21. It is good to create a contrast between the color of the face and the color of the neck.

   _____ True

   _____ False

22. How should foundation be applied?

   _____

23. How should you remove liquid foundation, tinted moisturizer and tube foundations from their containers?

   _____ a) with fingers
   _____ b) with a spatula
   _____ c) with a spoon
   _____ d) with a cotton ball

24. How are these foundations applied to the face?

   _____ a) with a comb
   _____ b) with a brush
   _____ c) with a sponge
   _____ d) with a washcloth

25. Powder and cream-to-powder foundation may be applied with a moist or dry _____.

26. Concealer is removed from the container with a _____ and may be applied with a concealer

   _____ or _____.

27. Once applied, what should you do with the concealer?

   _____

28. Concealer color should be:

    _____ a) darker than the skin color
    _____ b) lighter than the skin color
    _____ c) opposite the skin color
    _____ d) same as the skin color

29. Concealer that is noticeably lighter than skin can _____ to a problem area such as

    dark circles.

30. If covering a blemish, match skin very closely so as not to _____ the blemish.

31. The principles that apply to choosing foundation colors also apply to concealer colors.

    _____ True

    _____ False

32. Face powders are available in a variety of _____ and in different _____.

33. Light and medium weight powders are best for _____.

34. Heavier weight powders are best for _____.

35. How should you select a shade for face powder?

    _____

36. What is translucent powder and why is it used?

    _____

37. When is face powder applied and how?

    _____

    _____

38. In what forms is face powder available?

    _____

39. When is pressed powder recommended?

    _____

40. When is loose powder recommended?

   _____

41. When is cheek color applied?

   _____

42. Cheek color is available in four forms:

   a) _____   c) _____

   b) _____   d) _____

43. _____ cheek color blends well and is suitable for all skin types.

44. _____ cheek colors resemble cream foundation and are generally preferred for dry

   and normal skin.

45. _____ cheek color imparts a matte finish and is the most widely used.

46. _____cheek color comes in a variety of shades and tints, and is used to add color and

   to contour the cheeks.

47. How are dry cheek and loose powder blushes applied?

   _____

48. Cheek color _____ the part of the face where it is applied.

   a) darkens

   b) lightens

   c) accents

   d) highlights

49. Where should cheek color be applied?

   _____

50. Cheek color should be applied in toward the nose beyond the center of the eye.

_____ True

_____ False

51. Cheek color should be kept above the _____ at the tip of the nose.

52. Cheek color should extend above the outer corner of the eye.

_____ True

_____ False

53. Cheek color should be applied in:

_____ a) a bright, round circle
_____ b) a dark, round circle
_____ c) a blended fashion so it fades softly into the foundation
_____ d) a blended fashion so it is noticeably on top of foundation

54. When selecting a lip color be guided by a sense of_____.

55. What should you take into account when determining if a lip color will look good on a client?

_____

_____

56. Can lip color be applied directly from its container?

_____

57. What should you use to apply lip color?

_____

_____

58. How should you line the lips?

_____

_____

_____

_____

59. _____ is a colored pencil used to outline the lips.

60. Why use lip liner?

a) _____

b) _____

61. Lip liner comes in _____ or _____ pencil forms and is available in a variety of finishes.

62. Some lip liners double as _____ for ease of application.

63. Lip liner is usually applied before lip color to ensure proper shape and definition of the lips.

_____ True

_____ False

64. How should you choose a lip liner shade?

_____

65. The liner color should not be _____ darker or brighter than the lip shade.

66. If a darker liner is desired you should:

_____ a) outline both of the lips only

_____ b) outline the bottom of the lip only

_____ c) outline the top of the lip only

_____ d) fill in most of the lip only

67. How do you sharpen the lip liner pencil?

_____

_____

68. When applied to the lids, _____ makes the eyes appear brighter and more expressive.

69. What effect is achieved by matching eye shadow to eye color?

_____

70. What effect is achieved by using an eye shadow color different from the eye color?

_____

71. What effect is achieved by using a darker shade of eye color?

    _____

72. What effect is achieved by using a lighter shade of eye color?

    _____

73. What is the basic rule to remember when selecting eye color?

    _____

    _____

74. Eye colors and shadows are available in what forms?

    a) _____   _____   c) _____

    b) _____   d) _____

75. Eye shadow colors are generally referred to as _____.

76. A _____ is lighter than the client's skin tone and may have any finish.

77. What do highlight colors do?

    _____

78. A lighter color will make an area appear:

    _____ a) smaller

    _____ b) larger

    _____ c) more blue

    _____ d) more brown

79. A _____ is generally a medium tone that is close to the client's skin tone.

80. A base color is generally used to _____.

81. Where is a base color generally applied?

    _____

82. A _____ is a color that is deeper and darker than the client's skin tone.

83. When do you use a contour color?

_____

84. How is eye shadow applied?

_____

_____

85. Where is eye color applied?

_____

86. Only one color may be used on the eyelid.

_____ True

_____ False

87. For a natural look choose eyeliner that is the _____.

88. For a more dramatic look choose an eyeliner that is _____.

89. You must have a steady hand and be sure that your client remains still to ensure a _____

when applying eyeliner.

90. To help with the application, sharpen the eyeliner pencil and wipe with a clean tissue before:

_____ a) every other use

_____ b) each use

_____ c) every third use

_____ d) each day

91. Where is eyeliner applied?

_____

92. How should you apply powder shadow liner?

_____

_____

93. To use an eyebrow pencil you should: _____

94. When selecting a color to apply to the eyebrows you should avoid _____

    _____ , such as pale blonde or silver hair with black eyebrows.

95. Mascara may be used on all the lashes, from the _____ corners.

96. How do you apply mascara?

    _____

    _____

97. After the application you should

    _____ a) re-use the wand
    _____ b) dispose of the wand
    _____ c) send the wand home with the client
    _____ d) ask the client to save the wand for the next makeup application

98. What is the most common injury with mascara application?

    _____

99. When should you begin applying mascara to clients?

    _____

100. _____ remove eye makeup.

101. Most eye makeup products are _____ , so plain soap and water is less effective

    for removal.

102. Eye makeup removers are either _____ or _____ .

103. Oil-based removers generally contain _____ with a small amount of fragrance added.

104. Water-based removers generally contain a water solution to which _____

    _____ have been added.

105. _____ is a heavy makeup used for theatrical purposes.

106. _____ or _____ is a shaped, solid mass applied to the face with a moistened

cosmetic sponge and is generally used to cover scars and pigmentation defects.

107. Makeup brushes may be made of _____ or _____ hair with wooden or metal

handles.

108. Match each of the following makeup implements with the way in which they are used.

_____ 1. a powder brush	A. to give lift and upward curl to the upper lashes
_____ 2. a blush brush	B. for ease of application of shadow to the eyebrows or shadow liner to the eyes
_____ 3. a concealer brush	C. to remove excess mascara on lashes or to comb brows into place
_____ 4. a lip brush	D. to apply liquid liner or shadow to the eyes
_____ 5. an eye shadow brush	E. to apply shadow, blend eyeliner, or remove unwanted makeup from the eyes or lips
_____ 6. an eyeliner brush	F. to apply powder cheek color
_____ 7. an angle brush	G. to apply concealer around the eyes or over blemishes
_____ 8. a lash and brow brush	H. to apply concealer or lip color
_____ 9. tweezers	I. to apply mascara to a client; and because it is disposable, to ensure proper hygiene
_____ 10. an eyelash curler	J. to remove excess facial hair
_____ 11. a makeup sponge	K. to apply shadow and lip color or to blend eyeliner; may be used to remove unwanted makeup from eyes or lips
_____ 12. powder or cotton puffs	L. to apply and blend foundation, cream or powder blush, powder, or concealer
_____ 13. mascara wand	M. to remove such makeup as lipstick, foundation, concealer, powder, blush, and shadow from their containers
_____ 14. a plastic or wooden spatula	N. to apply and blend powder, powder foundation, or powder blush

_____15. disposable lip brush

_____16. sponge-tipped shadow applicator

_____17. cotton swabs

_____18. cotton pads or puffs

_____19. a pencil sharpener

O. to apply astringents or makeup removers; also used to apply powder products

P. to hygienically apply lip color to a a client

Q. to sharpen pencils prior to the application of eye or lip liner and to ensure hygienic application

R. to apply eye shadow color, to diffuse eye shadow color, and to blend eye shadow

S. to apply powder or blush and for blending edges of color

MAKEUP COLOR THEORY

109. What must you first determine before you choose eye, cheek, and lip colors for a client?

_____

110. If you select makeup shades that complement the client's skin color in level, what type of effect will you achieve?

_____

111. If you select makeup shades that contrast with the client's skin color, what type of effect will you achieve?

_____

112. Most skin tones and levels can wear a surprisingly large range of eye, cheek, and lip colors.

_____ True

_____ False

113. If skin color is _____ , you may use light colors for a soft, natural look.

114. Using medium to dark colors on light colored skin will create a more _____ look.

115. If skin color is _____ , medium tones will create an understated look.

116. Light or dark tones on a medium skin tone will provide more _____

and will appear _____ .

117. If skin color is _____ , dark tones will be most subtle.

118. Medium to light tones on a dark skin tone will be_____.

119. What caution should you remember when choosing tones lighter than the skin?

_____

120. If choosing light colors what is best to look for?

_____

121. What family of shades is the safest choice for eye, cheek and lip colors?_____

122. Why are neutrals a safe choice for everyone?

_____

_____

123. What are the most commonly used variations of neutral tones for eye shadows?

_____

124. What base color do browns have?

_____

_____

125. Charcoal gray is a_____.

126. Matching eye color with shadow color is the best way to enhance the eyes.

_____ True

_____ False

127. By contrasting eye color with_____colors, you emphasize the color most effectively.

128. What tool can you use to determine the complementary colors if you are not sure?

_____

129. What is the complementary color for blue eyes?

_____

130. Since the color orange contains yellow and red, are these also complementary colors for blue eyes?

_____

131. What are some common eye shadow color choices for blue eyes?

_____

_____

132. What is the complementary color for green eyes?

_____

133. Are red eye shadows considered attractive?

_____

134. What shades of reds are recommended to complement green eyes?

_____

135. What are some common eye color choices for green eyes?

_____

136. What is the complementary color for brown eyes?

_____

137. What colors would you recommended for a dramatic, contrasting look?

_____

138. When should you choose cheek and lip makeup colors?

_____

139. Is it important for the colors to coordinate?

_____

140. Name the tones that best coordinates with each of the following eye makeup colors.

_____ 1. Purple eye shadow	A.	cool tones
_____ 2. Gold eye shadow	B.	cool tones
_____ 3. Burgundy eye shadow	C.	warm tones
_____ 4. Silver eye shadow	D.	warm tones
_____ 5. Caramel eye shadow	E.	cool tones

141. _____ needs to be taken into account when determining eye makeup color.

142. Why is it important to take hair color into account when selecting eye color?

_____

143. In the spaces below, note the base tones in these hair colors.

_____	1.	warm blonde hair	A.	white-blonde, ash
_____	2.	cool blonde hair	B.	violet, blue
_____	3.	warm Red hair	C.	red-violet, violet
_____	4.	cool Red hair	D.	yellow, orange
_____	5.	warm Brown hair	E.	ash
_____	6.	cool Brown hair	F.	yellow, gold, orange
_____	7.	warm dark brown/black hair	G.	gold, copper, orange, red
_____	8.	cool dark brown/black hair	H.	copper, red

144. List the steps involved in selecting the right color tones for your client.

a) _____

b) _____

c) _____

d) _____

e) _____

f) _____

g) _____

h) _____

PROFESSIONAL MAKEUP APPLICATION

145. List the equipment, implements and materials needed to cleanse the skin before makeup application.

a) _____   c) _____

b) _____   d) _____

146. List the equipment, implements and materials needed for a makeup application.

_____

_____

147. List all of the accessory items needed for a makeup application.

_____

_____

_____

148. List all of the disposable tools or implements needed for a makeup application.

_____

_____

149. Before applying makeup you must have a client consultation.

_____ True

_____ False

150. Once the consultation is completed and before you touch the client you will need to _____.

151. When draping the client it is important to use a _____ or _____ to keep the hair out of the face.

152. Before applying makeup be sure to _____the face.

153. How should you apply cleansing cream or lotion to the face?

_____

_____

_____

_____

154. How should you remove the cleanser from the face?

_____

155. If makeup or color is particularly heavy in the eye or lip area, what should you do?

_____

156. After cleansing oily skin, apply an _____ before the makeup.

157. After cleansing dry skin, apply a _____ before the makeup.

158. The best way to apply a skin toner or astringent is to: _____

_____

_____

159. If the client has dry and delicate skin, apply a _____.

160. To apply a moisturizing lotion: _____

_____

161. Before applying any cosmetics you should groom the _____, removing any stray hairs by

tweezing the hair in the same direction in which it grows.

162. The first step in the makeup application is to_____.

163. To test the color you should blend the foundation on the client's _____.

164. Once you've selected the color, where should you place the foundation of application?

_____

165. What's the best way to apply foundation?

_____

_____

166. Where should you begin to blend the foundation?

_____

_____

167. If you need to apply concealer, how should that be accomplished?

_____

_____

168. If a powder foundation is used, the concealer must be applied _____ the foundation.

169. Concealer is commonly used _____.

170. After concealer, apply _____ .

171. What should you use to apply the powder and how should it be applied?

   _____

   _____

172. Why would you use a moistened cosmetic sponge over the finished makeup?

   _____

173. The first color cosmetic to be applied is the _____ .

174. Select a _____ color in a medium tone and then, beginning at the _____

   or _____ , apply lightly and blend outward with a brush or disposable applicator.

175. After shadow is applied select the _____ , which should harmonize with the mascara you

   will be applying.

176. To apply eyeliner, you should _____

   _____ .

177. Where can you apply eyeliner?

   _____

178. How should the eyebrows be groomed?

   _____

   _____

179. Where should mascara be applied?

   _____

   _____

180. When should cheek color be applied?

   _____

181. How should you determine where to put the blush?

_____

_____

182. If you are using powder cheek color, when and how is it applied?

_____

_____

183. How should the lips be lined?

_____

_____

_____

_____

_____

184. To remove the lip color from the container, use a _____ and then use a _____

to apply it to the lips.

185. What should you do to steady your hand?

_____

186. How should the client hold her lips while you are applying color?

_____

187. Once applied, ask the client to _____

_____.

188. How should you complete the lip color application?

_____

189. Once the makeup application is competed how should you clean up?

a) _____

b) _____

c) _____

d) _____

e) _____

f) _____

190. What is special-occasion makeup?

_____

191. What are some examples of special occasion makeup?

_____

192. Special occasions often come with special conditions such as the need for _____

_____ .

193. You may also add drama by applying false _____ and using _____

colors on the eyes, lips, cheeks, or complexion.

194. Makeup for photography should be _____ , since shimmer may reflect light too much.

195. To create a striking contour to eyes do the following.

a) _____

_____

b) _____

_____

c) _____

_____

d) _____

_____

e) _____

f) _____

_____

g) _____

_____

196. To create dramatic smoky eyes do the following.

a) _____

_____

b) _____

_____

c) _____

_____

d) _____

_____

e) _____

_____

f) _____

_____

g) _____

_____

197. To create a special occasion look for cheeks, try either of the following.

a) _____

_____

b) _____

_____

198. To create a special occasion look for lips, do the following

    a) _____

    b) _____

    c) _____

CORRECTIVE MAKEUP

199. What are some of the most common facial flaws?

    a) _____

    b) _____

    c) _____

200. Facial makeup can create the illusion of better_____ and _____ when so desired.

201. Facial features can be accented with proper_____ , subdued with correct _____ ,

    and balanced with the proper _____ .

202. A basic rule for the application of makeup is that highlighting_____ a feature, while

    shadowing_____ it.

203. A highlight is produced when a cosmetic, usually foundation that is _____

    _____ , is used on a particular part of the face.

204. A shadow is formed when the foundation is _____ .

205. The use of shadows minimizes _____features so that they are less noticeable.

206. What is the first step in undertaking any kind of corrective makeup application?

    _____

207. What is the basic goal of all makeup application?

    _____

208. What face shape is considered well-proportioned and ideal?

    _____

209. What is the goal of an effective makeup application?

_____

210. Why is the oval face shape considered ideal?

_____

_____

211. The face is divided into three equal _____ sections.

212. The first third is measured from the _____ to the _____.

213. The second third is measured from the _____ to _____.

214. The last third is measured from the _____ to _____.

215. The _____ face is usually broader in proportion to its length than the oval face with a rounding

chin and hairline.

216. Corrective makeup can be applied to _____ and _____ the round face.

217. The _____ face is composed of comparatively straight lines with a wide forehead

and square jawline.

218. Corrective makeup can be applied to offset the _____ and _____ the hard lines

around a square face.

219. A jaw that is wider than the forehead characterizes the _____ face.

220. Corrective makeup can be applied to create _____ at the forehead, _____

the jaw line, and add _____ to the face.

221. The _____ face has a wide forehead and narrow, pointed chin.

222. Corrective makeup can be applied to minimize the width of the _____ and to increase the

width of the _____.

223. The _____ face has a narrow forehead with the greatest width across
the cheekbones.

224. Corrective makeup can be applied to _____ the width across the cheekbone line.

225. The _____ face has greater length in proportion to its width than the square or round
face and is long and narrow.

226. Corrective makeup can be applied to create the illusion of _____ across the cheekbone line,
making the face appear _____.

227. For a _____ forehead, the application of a lighter foundation lends a broader appearance between
the brows and hairline.

228. For a _____ forehead, apply a darker foundation over the prominent area to give an
illusion of fullness to the rest of the face and minimize the bulge.

229. Can a change in hairstyle help camouflage a problem forehead?

_____

230. For a _____ , apply a darker foundation on the nose and a lighter
foundation on the cheeks at the sides of the nose.

231. What effect will this give?

_____

232. Should you place cheek color close to the nose?

_____

233. For a _____ , apply a lighter foundation down the center of the nose,
ending at the tip.

234. What effect will this have?

_____

235. If the nostrils are wide, what should you do?

_____

236. For a _____, use a darker foundation on the sides of the nose and nostrils.

237. When using a dark tone foundation to be sure to carefully blend it to avoid_____.

238. For a _____and_____, shadow the chin with a darker

    foundation and highlight the nose with a lighter foundation.

239. For a _____, highlight the chin by using a lighter foundation than the one used

    on the face.

240. For a _____, use a darker foundation on the sagging portion, and use a natural

    skin tone foundation on the face.

241. When applying makeup, how should the neck be treated?

    a) ignore it

    b) blend it

    c) darken it

    d) lighten it

242. How should you set makeup on the neck?

_____

243. To correct a _____, apply a darker shade of foundation over the heavy area of the jaw,

    starting at the temples.

244. What effect will this have?

_____

245. To correct a _____jawline, highlight it by using a lighter foundation shade.

246. For a _____, _____, or_____ face, apply a darker shade of

    foundation over the prominent part of the jawline.

247. What effect will this have?

_____

_____

248. For a _____ and a _____ neck, use a darker foundation on the neck than the one used on the face.

249. What effect will this have?

_____

250. For a _____ , apply a lighter shade of foundation on the neck than the one used on the face.

251. What effect will this have?

_____

252. _____ can be lengthened by extending eye shadow beyond the outer corner of the eyes.

253. _____ are closer together than the length of one eye.

254. For eyes that are too close together, lightly apply shadow up from the _____.

255. _____ eyes can be minimized by blending the shadow carefully over the prominent part of the upper lid, carrying it lightly toward the eyebrow, using a medium-deep shadow color.

256. To correct _____ shadow evenly and lightly across the lid from the edge of the eyelash line to the small crease in the eye socket.

257. To make _____ eyes appear larger, extend the shadow slightly above, beyond and below the eyes.

258. For _____ eyes, apply the shadow on the upper inner side of the eyelid, toward the nose, and blend carefully.

259. Use bright, light, reflective colors and use the lightest color in the crease, and a light to medium color sparingly on the lid and brow bone to correct _____ .

260. To correct _____ apply concealer over the dark area, blending and smoothing

it into the surrounding area.

261. The eyebrow is the _____ for the eye, and overgrown eyebrows can cast a _____

on the brow bone or between the two eyebrows.

262. _____ eyebrows can make the face look puffy or protruding, or may give the eyes a

surprised look.

263. Ideally, where should the eyebrow begin?

_____

264. The second line to determine the ideal eyebrow shape is drawn at an angle from the _____

_____ .

265. The third line is vertical, from the _____ .

266. What should you do if the arch is too high?

_____

_____

267. If a person has a low forehead she should wear a _____ because it gives more height to a

very low forehead.

268. If a person has wide-set eyes you should extend the eyebrow lines to the _____

of the eyes.

269. If a person has close-set eyes, you should _____ the distance between the eyebrows and

slightly extend them outward.

270. If a person has a round face you should arch the brows _____ to make the face appear narrower.

271. If a person has a long face she should make the eyebrows almost _____ to create the illusion

of a shorter face.

272. If a person has a square face she should wear a _____ arch on the ends of the eyebrows.

273. What can you do for a client who has ruddy skin?

_____

274. What can you do for a client who has sallow skin?

_____

275. Age lines and wrinkles due to dry skin can be minimized with _____ .

ARTIFICIAL EYELASHES

276. Who uses false eyelashes?

_____

277. _____ are eyelash hairs on a strip that are applied with adhesive to the natural lash line.

278. _____ are separate artificial eyelashes that are applied to the eyelids one at a time.

279. _____ is the product used to make artificial eyelashes adhere, or stick, to the

natural lash line.

280. List all of the implements and materials needed to apply band lashes.

_____

_____

_____

_____

281. How should you prepare for applying band lashes?

a) _____

_____

b) _____

c) _____

d) _____

e) _____

f) _____

282. Describe the procedure for applying band lashes.

a) _____

b) _____

c) _____

_____

d) _____

e) _____

f) _____

_____

_____

g) _____

283. Describe the cleanup process.

a) _____

b) _____

c) _____

d) _____

e) _____

f) _____

284. How should band eyelashes be removed?

_____

285. Starting from the _____ , remove the lashes carefully to avoid pulling out the

client's own lashes.

286. Individual eyelashes attach directly to a _____ .

287. How long do individual eyelashes last?

_____

21

NAIL STRUCTURE AND GROWTH

See Milady's Standard Cosmetology Theory Workbook

22
MANICURING AND PEDICURING

Date: _____

Rating: _____

Text Pages: 757-793

POINT TO PONDER:

"Getting an idea should be like sitting down on a pin; it should make you jump up and do something."—E.L. Simpson

1. In ancient times, those who wore long, polished, and tinted fingernails were considered _____.

2. _____ and _____ make up one of the biggest growth areas in salon services today.

3. What is the derivation of the word "manicure"?

   _____

   _____

4. What is the derivation of the word pedicure?

   _____

5. To practice as a professional nail technician, you should have an understanding of the following.

   a) _____

   _____

   b) _____

   _____

   c) _____

   _____

   d) _____

   _____

   e) _____

   _____

f) _____

_____

NAIL CARE TOOLS

6. The four basic categories of nail tools are

_____

7. _____ consists of the permanent tools you will be using to perform nail services.

8. List the equipment you will need to use in nail care.

a) _____   e) _____

b) _____   f) _____

c) _____   g) _____

d) _____   h) _____

9. What are implements?

_____

_____

10. Match the following implements with their use in nail care.

_____ 1. cuticle nipper   A. implement used to shorten nails
_____ 2. cuticle pusher   B. metal instrument used to file and shape the nails
_____ 3. emery board   C. implement used to lift small bits of cuticle from the nail
_____ 4. nail brush   D. implement used to loosen and push back the cuticle around
                                    nails
_____ 5. nail buffer   E. small brush used to clean under and around the nails
_____ 6. nail clippers   F. used to loosen the cuticle around the base of the nail or to
                                    clean under the free edge
_____ 7. nail file   G. instrument with rough ridges, used for shaping and
                                    smoothing nails
_____ 8. orangewood stick   H. instrument used with a polishing powder to polish the nails
                                    to a high luster
_____ 9. tweezers   I. small cutting tool used to nip or cut excess cuticle at the base
                                    of the nail

11. Next to each implement below note whether it can be reused or must be discarded after each client.

cuticle nipper _____

cuticle pusher _____

emery board _____

nail brush _____

nail buffer _____

nail clippers _____

nail file _____

orangewood stick _____

tweezers _____

12. How many sets of metal implements should you have at any time and why?

_____

_____

13. How long does it take to sanitize implements?

_____

14. What are the steps to follow for proper sanitation?

a) _____

_____

b) _____

_____

c) _____

_____

d) _____

_____

15. What is a nail cosmetic?

_____

16. What is an antiseptic used for?

_____

17. What is a base coat?

_____

_____

_____

18. What is cuticle cream?

_____

_____

19. What is cuticle oil?

_____

20. What is cuticle remover or solvent?

_____

_____

21. What is dry nail polish?

_____

22. What are hand creams and lotions?

_____

_____

_____

23. What is liquid nail polish or lacquer?

_____

24. What is nail bleach?

_____

25. What is nail conditioner?

_____

_____

26. What is nail dryer?

_____

_____

27. What is nail hardener or strengthener?

_____

_____

28. What is polish remover and when do you use it?

_____

29. What is polish thinner?

_____

30. What is top coat or sealer?

_____

_____

31. In addition to making the finished nail look attractive, what other purpose does nail polish serve?

_____

32. Name the three types of nail hardeners or strengtheners.

    a) _____   c) _____

    b) _____

33. _____ utilize keratin fibers to strengthen the nail.

34. _____ are a combination of clear polish and nylon fibers, applied first

vertically, then horizontally on the nail plate.

35. _____ are a combination of clear polish and a protein such as collagen.

36. To offset the drying action of nail polish removers, _____ is frequently in the solution.

37. When would you opt to use non-acetone polish remover? Why?

_____

_____

38. List the materials that are used during a service but must be replaced for each client.

a) _____

b) _____

c) _____

d) _____

e) _____

f) _____

g) _____

h) _____

i) _____

j) _____

39. What type of trash container should be used and how often should it be emptied?

_____

_____

40. What is aluminum salt and what is it used for?

_____

THE MANICURE TABLE

41. Keeping a neat manicure table makes clients feel _____ .

42. When giving a professional manicure, seat the next client and then quickly clean up your manicure table.

_____ True

_____ False

43. The best time to clear the manicure table is at the end of the day.

_____ True

_____ False

44. In preparation for giving a manicure, you should wash table and drawer with a warm, sudsy solution.

_____ True

_____ False

45. You should always place a clean or disposable towel over the client's cushion.

_____ True

_____ False

46. Where should you place a bowl of warm, soapy water? _____

47. If you are giving a hot oil manicure, what replaces the fingerbowl and brush?

_____

48. Where should disinfected metal implements and a new orangewood stick be placed?

_____

49. Where should cream or lotion bottles and nail polishes be arranged and how?

_____

50. Where should the disinfected abrasive and fresh emery boards be placed?

_____

51. A small plastic bag should be attached to the manicure table with adhesive tape, on either the right or left side, for waste materials.

_____ True

_____ False

52. A fresh disinfectant solution should be prepared for your implements on a daily basis.

_____ True

_____ False

CLIENT CONSULTATION

53. What must you do before servicing any nail or pedicure client?

_____

54. What things should you discuss during the consultation?

_____

_____

55. What should you do if the client has a nail or skin disorder that prevents you from performing a service?

_____

_____

56. What are the two parts of a consultation?

_____

57. What is the analysis portion of the consultation?

_____

_____

_____

_____

58. What is the "recommendations" portion of the consultation?

_____

_____

59. To perform a useful consultation, you will need to

a) _____

b) _____

c) _____

d) _____

60. A well-handled consultation demonstrates _____

_____.

61. Should you ask questions concerning the client's health? Why?

_____

_____

62. Before you begin to work on a client's nails, both you and the client should agree on which nail

_____ is desired.

63. The five general nail shapes are

a) _____   d) _____

b) _____   e) _____

c) _____

64. What things should you be mindful of when deciding which shape to go with?

a) _____   c) _____

b) _____   d) _____

65. It is generally felt that nails should be shaped to mirror the shape of the _____ .

66. People who perform work with their hands usually require _____ nails in order to

avoid nail breakage and injury.

67. The _____ nail shape is completely straight across the free edge with no rounding at the edges.

68. The _____ nail shape should extend only slightly past the tip of the finger with the nail tip

rounded off.

69. How should a round nail shape be polished?

_____

_____

70. The _____ nail shape is the ideal nail shape and can be styled by covering the entire nail with

polish, leaving the free edge white, or leaving the half moon at the base of the nail white.

71. The _____ nail shape is well suited for the thin, delicate hand.

72. The _____ nail shape is a square nail with the ends rounded or taken off.

73. What shapes combine to create "squoval"?

_____

THE PLAIN MANICURE

74. As a professional nail technician, you will follow a _____ procedure for all services you

    perform.

     a) two-part

     b) three-part

     c) four-part

     d) five-part

75. The three part sequence includes _____

    _____.

76. What eight steps must be completed in the pre-service portion of the manicure?

     a) _____

    _____

     b) _____

    _____

     c) _____

    _____

     d) _____

    _____

     e) _____

    _____

     f) _____

    _____

     g) _____

    _____

     h) _____

    _____

77. During the actual manicure procedure, what things should you discuss with your client?

_____

_____

78. Why would you ask clients to replace jewelry, locate keys, pay for the service as well as any retail products, and put on any outer clothing such as sweaters or jackets before polishing the nails?

_____

79. The manicure post-service includes

a) _____

_____

b) _____

_____

c) _____

_____

d) _____

_____

e) _____

_____

80. What is the purpose of giving a hand massage with each manicure?

_____

81. During a hand massage, and while you are holding the client's hand, where should you place a dab of hand lotion?

_____

82. What type of action should you take to help limber the client's wrist?

_____

83. How should you massage and relax the hand?

_____

_____

84. How should you massage the wrist?

_____

_____

85. How should you finish the massage?

_____

_____

86. Describe the procedure for massaging the forearm and elbow.

a) _____

_____

b) _____

_____

_____

c) _____

_____

d) _____

_____

e) _____

_____

f) _____

_____

g) _____

_____

87. To provide a plain manicure, you will need.

_____ a)   some of your basic implements and materials
_____ b)   most of your basic implements and materials
_____ c)   all of your basic implements and materials
_____ d)   none of your basic implements and materials

88. The first step in giving the plain manicure is to _____

_____

89. How should old polish be removed?

_____

_____

_____

90. After polish is completely removed, you should: _____ .

91. How do you decide what shape the nails should be?

_____

92. On which finger do you begin to file the nails?

_____

93. If nails need shortening, they can be cut with

_____ a) cuticle nippers

_____ b) orangewood stick

_____ c) fingernail clippers

_____ d) emery board

94. To soften the cuticle you should _____ .

95. Should you immerse both hands into the finger bowl at one time to soften cuticles?

_____

_____

96. Once the cuticles have been softened how should you clean the nails?

_____

_____

97. How should you dry the fingertips?

_____

_____

98. How should you prepare the orangewood stick to push back the cuticles?

_____

_____

_____

99. What kind of movement of the orangewood stick helps you to remove cuticle that clings to the nail plate?

_____

100. How should you clean under the free edge?

_____

_____

101. If it is necessary to bleach under the free edge, how is that accomplished?

_____

_____

102. Once the cuticles are shaped, what should be applied?

_____

_____

103. After the left hand is completed, what should you do?

_____

_____

104. Once both hands are completed, what should you do?

_____

_____

105. To remove any remaining pieces of cuticle you should _____

_____.

106. When should a hand or hand/arm massage be given with a plain manicure?

_____

107. How should base coat be applied?

_____

_____

108. How do you know when the base coat is dry? _____

109. If using a nail strengthener/hardener, when is it applied? _____

110. When is colored polish applied? _____

111. How do you apply colored polish?

_____

_____

_____

112. If you miss a small area on the nail, you can _____ .

113. How can you remove excess polish?

_____

_____

114. After two coats of polish, what should you apply next?

_____

_____

115. If you us a UV top coat, place both the client's hands under _____ .

116. Why would you use instant nail dry?

_____

117. A fringe of loose skin left around the nail after a manicure can be caused by: _____

_____ .

118. Callus growth at the fingertips can be softened by the application of _____ .

119. Gentle rubbing with _____ or an abrasive is also a good way to begin the process of

removing calluses.

120. Stains on fingernails may be bleached with prepared nail bleach or _____ .

121. What other way can stains be removed?

_____

OTHER TYPES OF MANICURES

122. A _____ is one in which a heated oil, cream, or lotion is applied to the cuticles to

soften them before pushing them back.

123. What kinds of nails and cuticles benefit from a hot oil manicure?

_____

124. What kind of oil should be used in a hot oil manicure?

_____

125. It is suggested that a reconditioning hot oil manicure be performed

_____ a)   once a day
_____ b)   once a week
_____ c)   once a month
_____ d)   once a year

126. Hot oil manicures are also beneficial for people who _____ because it helps keep

rough cuticles soft.

127. Preheat the oil for _____ minutes.

a)   5

b)   10

c)   15

d)   20

128. To give a hot oil manicure, perform a plain manicure to the point at which you would: _____

_____ .

129. Place the hands in the heated oil and _____.

130. Massage the hands and wrists _____.

131. To remove oil,_____ before applying

the base coat.

132. A _____ is a manicure in which the free edge of the nail is polished, tipped, or

sculpted in an opaque color while the nail plate is polished or left a more translucent color.

133. A French manicure usually uses a dramatic _____ on the free edge of the nail, whereas

the American manicure calls for a _____.

134. List the procedure for a French manicure.

a) _____

_____

b) _____

_____

c) _____

_____

d) _____

_____

e) _____

_____

f) _____

_____

g) _____

_____

h) _____

_____

135. If the nail has pitting, lines, or ridges, use a _____.

136. What shape nails should men choose?

_____

137. You can apply a _____ instead of a liquid polish for a man's manicure.

138. For a man's manicure follow the same procedure for a plain manicure up to _____

_____.

139. How should you buff the nails during a man's manicure?

_____

_____

140. To prevent a hot or burning sensation, lift the buffer from the nail after _____.

_____ a) each stroke
_____ b) every other stroke
_____ c) every tenth stroke
_____ d) every twentieth stroke

141. What effect does buffing have?

_____

_____

142. How should you finish a man's manicure

a) _____

b) _____

c) _____

143. What is a booth manicure?

_____

_____

144. What is an electric manicure?

_____

_____

PEDICURES

145. _____ has become an important salon service because of popular shoe

styles that expose the heels and toes.

146. When are pedicures in greatest demand?

_____

_____

147. When making a pedicure appointment, suggest that the client wear _____ shoes or

_____ so that the polish will not smear.

148. An alternative the salon can offer to open-toed shoes is be to provide _____

along with _____ to keep those toes warm in colder weather.

149. In addition to the equipment, implements, and materials used for manicuring, pedicuring requires:

a) _____

b) _____

c) _____

d) _____

e) _____

f) _____

g) _____

h) _____

i) _____

j) _____

k) _____

l) _____

m) _____

n) _____

o) _____

p) _____

q) _____

r) _____

s) _____

t) _____

u) _____

150. What is a curette and what is it used for?

_____

_____

151. What is a nail rasp and what is it used for?

_____

_____

152. What is a diamond nail file and what is it used for?

_____

153. What is a foot file or paddle?

_____

154. Too light a touch or hold while performing a foot massage will produce a _____,

which is not relaxing for most clients.

155. Match these illustrations for the massage with their correct descriptions:

   A. percussion or tapotement movement

   B. relaxer movement to the joints of
   the foot

   C. fist twist compression

   D. joint movement for toes

   E. effleurage (light or hard stroking
   movements) on top of the foot

   F. effleurage movement on toes

   G. effleurage on the heel (bottom of
   foot)

   H. metatarsal scissors

   I. thumb compression (friction movement)

   _____ 1.   _____ 2.   _____ 3.

   _____ 4.   _____ 5.   _____ 6.

   _____ 7.   _____ 8.   _____ 9.

156. How far up the leg may the foot massage be extended?

   _____

157. On the calf area of the leg, you may use _____ movements up to the backside of the knee.

158. Describe the steps of the pedicure preparation or pre-service

   a) _____

   _____

   b) _____

   _____

c) _____

_____

d) _____

_____

e) _____

_____

f) _____

_____

g) _____

_____

h) _____

_____

i) _____

_____

j) _____

_____

159. During the actual pedicure procedure, what should you discuss with your client?

_____

_____

160. The first step in the pedicure process is to _____ .

161. If clipping the toenails, clip the nails of the _____ foot first, taking care that they are even with the end of the toe.

162. _____ are inserted between the toes of the feet prior to _____ .

163. How should toenails be filed?

_____

_____

164. Where should you use a foot file?

_____

165. After filing, what is the next step?

_____

166. When the left foot is soaking, you should _____ .

167. Once the right foot is soaking, you should _____

_____ .

168. With a new cotton-tipped orangewood stick, apply _____ to the cuticle and under

the free edge of each toenail of the left foot.

169. _____ the cuticle gently with the cotton-tipped orangewood stick, keeping the cuticle

moist with additional lotion or water.

170. Should you cut the cuticle while giving a pedicure?

_____

171. After the foot has been rinsed and dried, apply _____ and massage the foot.

172. Once the massage is completed, place the foot:

_____ a)　in the basin
_____ b)　on a clean towel on the floor
_____ c)　in a pedicure slipper
_____ d)　in a shoe

173. Before applying the base coat be sure to remove traces of _____ from the toenails.

174. To polish toenails apply _____ .

SAFETY RULES IN MANICURING AND PEDICURING

175. What is the procedure for handling blood spills?

a) _____

_____

_____

b) _____

_____

_____

c) _____

_____

_____

d) _____

_____

_____

e) _____

_____

_____

f) _____

_____

_____

g) _____

_____

_____

h) _____

_____

_____

23

ADVANCED NAIL TECHNIQUES

Date: _____

Rating: _____

Text Pages: 795-824

POINT TO PONDER:

"He is great who can do what he wishes; he is wise who wishes to do what he can."—August Iffland

1. What are some solutions for clients who want to wear long nails but who have a problem growing natural nails to the length and strength desired?

a) _____   d) _____

b) _____   e) _____

c) _____

2. Artificial nails can be used for the following purposes:

a) _____

b) _____

c) _____

d) _____

PRE-SERVICE AND POST-SERVICE PROCEDURES

3. The artificial nail service, like other services, should begin with a _____ .

4. The most important issue you and your client will determine is the type of nail service best suited to her _____ .

5. The pre-service procedure consists of the following steps:

a) _____

b) _____

_____

c) _____

_____

d) _____

e) _____

_____

f) _____

_____

g) _____

h) _____

i) _____

j) _____

k) _____

l) _____

m) _____

n) _____

_____

6. After the service you will want to _____ with your client in order to maintain his or her nails according to the prescribed maintenance schedule.

7. What are some retail products you could offer that will help your client take care of her nails between appointments?

_____

8. How should you clean your table and the surrounding area?

_____

_____

NAIL TIPS

9. The addition of pre-formed artificial nails applied to the tips of the natural fingernails is a service called

    _____ .

10. What are nail tips commonly made of and why are they used?

    _____

11. Usually tips are combined with another artificial nail service, such as _____ .

12. A wrap, acrylic, or gel applied over the entire natural nail plate is called an _____ .

13. Nail tips are secured to the natural nails with _____ or _____ .

14. These agents come in either a _____ or a

    _____ , or as a _____ .

15. The _____ is the point where the nail plate meets the tip before it is glued to the nail.

16. The tip should never cover more than:

    _____ a) $\frac{1}{3}$ of the natural nail plate

    _____ b) $\frac{1}{2}$ of the natural nail plate

    _____ c) $\frac{3}{4}$ of the natural nail plate

    _____ d) $\frac{3}{8}$ of the natural nail plate

17. Nail tips should be pre-beveled along the edge closest to the (cuticle) to thin out the plastic.

    _____ a) free edge

    _____ b) cuticle

    _____ c) sides

    _____ d) half moon

18. Why are pre-beveled tips useful?

    _____

    _____

19. Be sure to fit each client with the precise _____ and _____ tip for her needs.

20. In addition to the materials on your basic manicuring table, you will need the following to apply tips:

    a) _____   d) _____

    b) _____   e) _____

    c) _____   f) _____

21. You should first _____, working from little

    finger to thumb.

22. Before applying nail tips be sure to push back the _____ .

23. Buff the natural nails to remove _____, then brush away the dust.

24. How do you know if you have selected the proper size tip?

    _____

    _____

25. What can you do if the well covers too much of the nail?

    _____

26. Apply _____ to remove the remaining natural oil and to dehydrate the nail for better

    adhesion.

27. Where should adhesive be applied?

    _____

28. How should adhesive be applied?

    _____

    _____

29. What is the "stop, rock, and hold" procedure?

    _____

    _____

30. How should you strengthen the stress point?

_____

31. How should you trim the nail tip to the desired length?

_____

32. How can you blend the tip into the natural nail?

_____

33. _____ the tip for a perfect blend between the natural nail plate and the tip extension.

34. After the nails have been buffed, you may _____ the nail.

35. After the tip is placed you may proceed with any other service such as _____.

36. Clients wearing tips will need _____ or _____ manicures to allow for regluing

    and rebuffing.

37. If a client is wearing temporary tips, you would reglue at the _____

    _____.

38. Most tips will require _____ polish remover, so as not to dissolve the tips.

39. How are nail tips removed?

_____

_____

_____

40. Prying tips off can be damaging to the nail _____.

41. Once the tip is removed, buff the nail with a _____ to remove any glue residue and

    condition the cuticle and surrounding skin with _____.

NAIL WRAPS

42. _____ is a corrective treatment that forms a protective coating for a damaged or fragile

    nail.

43. Nail wraps can be applied over the natural nail or over a set of tips.

    _____ True

    _____ False

44. List the materials commonly used in nail wraps:

    _____   _____

    _____   _____

45. Match the nail wrap with its description.

    _____ 1. silk   A. very thin paper that dissolves in both any type of polish remover;
                                   considered temporary

    _____ 2. fiberglass   B. coarse material that provides a durable wrap; requires a colored
                                   polish to cover the completed nail

    _____ 3. linen   C. gives a smooth, even appearance to the nail, becomes almost
                                   transparent when adhesive is applied

    _____ 4. paper   D. a thin synthetic mesh with a loose weave; strong and durable

46. In addition to the materials on your basic manicuring table, you will need the following to complete a
    nail wrap service:

    a) _____

    b) _____

    c) _____

    d) _____

    e) _____

    f) _____

    g) _____

47. What steps should you take to prepare for nail wraps?

    a) _____

    b) _____

c) _____

d) _____

e) _____

48. List the steps involved in applying nail wraps:

a) _____

b) _____

c) _____

d) _____

e) _____

f) _____

g) _____

h) _____

i) _____

j) _____

k) _____

_____

l) _____

49. How are nail wraps removed?

_____

_____

_____

_____

50. How are fabric wraps maintained?

_____

51. What steps do you follow for the two-week maintenance?

a) _____

b) _____

c) _____

d) _____

_____

e) _____

f) _____

g) _____

h) _____

i) _____

j) _____

52. What steps do you follow for the four-week maintenance?

a) _____

b) _____

c) _____

d) _____

_____

e) _____

f) _____

g) _____

h) _____

i) _____

j) _____

k) _____

l) _____

53. What can be done to strengthen a weak point or repair a break in the nail?

_____

54. A _____ is a strip of fabric cut to $\frac{1}{8}$ inch and applied to the weak point of the nail using the four-week maintenance procedure.

55. A _____ is a piece of fabric that is cut to completely cover the crack or break in the nail.

56. _____ is a polish made with tiny fibers designed to strengthen and preserve the natural nail as it grows.

57. How is a liquid nail wrap used?

_____

_____

ACRYLIC NAILS

58. _____ nails, often referred to as sculptured nails, are artificial nails that are created by combining a liquid acrylic product with a powdered product.

59. How are acrylic nails applied?

_____

_____

60. For what purposes are acrylics used?

_____

61. What are the three basic ingredients in the acrylic nail process?

a) _____   c) _____

b) _____

62. A _____ is a substance made up of many small molecules that are not attached to one another.

63. A _____ is a hard substance formed by combining many small molecules, usually in a long chain-like structure.

64. A polymer is a liquid.

_____ True

_____ False

65. A _____ is any substance having the power to increase the velocity (speed) of a chemical

reaction.

66. Powdered acrylic is a combination of ground-up _____ and a _____ .

67. What is curing?

_____

_____

68. Nail forms are made of _____

_____ .

69. A _____ is a substance that improves adhesion, or attachment, and prepares the nail surface for

bonding with the acrylic material.

70. An Acid primer is widely used to help _____ the acrylic to the natural nail.

71. A _____ is noninvasive to the natural nail and not corrosive on the skin but may

not be as effective as acid primer.

72. How much primer should be applied? What happens if you apply too much primer?

_____

73. What happens of nails are overly primed?

_____

74. What color is primer when dry?

_____ a) yellow
_____ b) clear
_____ c) pink
_____ d) white

75. In addition to the materials on your basic manicuring table, you will need the following to apply acrylic over nails:

a) _____   f) _____

b) _____   g) _____

c) _____   h) _____

d) _____   i) _____

e) _____

76. What is the procedure for applying acrylic over nails?

a) _____

b) _____

c) _____

d) _____

e) _____

f) _____

g) _____

h) _____

_____

i) _____

j) _____

_____

k) _____

_____

l) _____

_____

_____

m) _____

n) _____

o) _____

p) _____

q) _____

77. Acrylic _____ are artificial nails that use the same acrylic material as sculptured nails but are

applied directly to the natural nail surface instead of being extended.

78. Why are these overlays useful?

_____

79. How are acrylic overlays applied?

_____

80. What is a fill?

_____

81. What is rebalancing?

_____

82. What is the procedure for applying acrylic nail fills?

a) _____

b) _____

c) _____

d) _____

_____

e) _____

f) _____

_____

g) _____

h) _____

i) _____

_____

j) _____

_____

k) _____

l) _____

83. If an acrylic nail is badly chipped or cracked, you should _____

_____ .

84. To remove an acrylic nail you should _____

_____ .

GELS

85. What are gel nails?

_____

86. How many types of gels are there?

_____

87. _____ harden when they are exposed to a special light source, either ultraviolet or

halogen.

88. _____ harden when an activator or accelerator is sprayed or brushed on, or when they

are soaked in water.

89. In addition to the materials on your basic manicuring table, you will need the following to apply light-cured gels:

a) _____   e) _____

b) _____   f) _____

c) _____   g) _____

d) _____   h) _____

90. Describe the procedure for applying light-cured gels.

a) _____

b) _____

c) _____

d) _____

e) _____

f) _____

g) _____

h) _____

i) _____

j) _____

k) _____

l) _____

m) _____

n) _____

o) _____

91. In addition to the materials on your basic manicuring table, you will need the following to apply no-light cured gels:

a) _____ e) _____

b) _____ f) _____

c) _____ g) _____

d) _____

92. Describe the procedure for applying no-light cured gel on nails:

a) _____

b) _____

c) _____

d) _____

_____

e) _____

f) _____

93. Both light-cured and non-light-cured gels should be maintained every _____ ,

   depending on how fast the client's nails grow.

   a) Five to six days

   b) Six to ten days

   c) One to two weeks

   d) Two to three weeks

94. How are gel nails removed?

   _____

   _____

DIPPED NAILS

95. Dipped nails are created by _____ .

96. Most dipped nails do not rely on an acrylic monomer but use instead a _____ , a very

   fast-setting glue which comes in different viscosities and can be applied in several ways.

97. What is the procedure for dipped nails?

   a) _____

   b) _____

   c) _____

   d) _____

NAIL ART

98. Who wears nail art?

   _____

99. What types of nail art are available?

    a) _____

       _____

    b) _____

    c) _____

    d) _____

       _____

    e) _____

       _____

    f) _____

       _____

24

THE SALON BUSINESS

See Milady's Standard Cosmetology Theory Workbook

25

SEEKING EMPLOYMENT

See Milady's Standard Cosmetology Theory Workbook

26

ON THE JOB

See Milady's Standard Cosmetology Theory Workbook